A Matter of Life

of Life

The Story of a Medical Breakthrough

Robert Edwards
Patrick Steptoe

Hutchinson
London Melbourne Sydney Auckland Johannesburg

Hutchinson & Co. (Publishers) Ltd

An imprint of the Hutchinson Publishing Group

3 Fitzroy Square, London W1P 6JD

Hutchinson Group (Australia) Pty Ltd
30-32 Cremorne Street, Richmond South, Victoria 3121
PO Box 151, Broadway, New South Wales 2007

Hutchinson Group (NZ) Ltd
32-34 View Road, PO Box 40-086, Glenfield, Auckland 10

Hutchinson Group (SA) (Pty) Ltd
PO Box 337, Bergvlei 2012, South Africa

First published 1980
© Finestride Ltd & Crownchime Ltd 1980

Set in APS 5 Saul by Brown, Knight & Truscott Ltd

Printed in Great Britain by The Anchor Press Ltd
and bound by Wm Brendon & Son Ltd
both of Tiptree, Essex

ISBN 0 09 139180 6

This book is dedicated
to our loyal staff,
to the patients who have contributed
so much to help us and each other,
and especially to
Dr Dannie Abse
with gratitude for his invaluable help
in preparing it for publication

Contents

Illustrations

1
The Quest

Patrick Steptoe

She did not realize I was a medical student. Despite my youthful appearance she called me, 'Doctor,' then briefly lost control 'What have I done wrong,' she cried, 'not to have a family of my own?' Perturbed I tried to comfort her and in a moment she managed to continue, 'I would have liked to have a large family but I've been married seven years and . . . .' Her voice trailed off.

I nodded. There were eight in my own family, eight brothers and sisters in the happy Steptoe family. I was the fifth and youngest son. 'I understand,' I said.

Gently I asked her more questions and finally said, 'Mr Gwillim will see you soon.'

C. M. Gwillim was the consultant at St George's Hospital in London. He was a superb gynaecologist and obstetrician and I was on his firm.

Soon the notes I had made, her case-history, lay on Mr Gwillim's desk. He read them out to the other medical students while I gazed beyond Mr Gwillim's head at the patient's tell-tale confirmatory X rays on the luminous screens. It was evident that she, like millions of other women all over the world, suffered from tubal occlusions, possibly as a result of some previous infection, and consequently she would never be able to conceive and have a baby. Her own ovum descending each month could not pass through her blocked Fallopian tubes to be fertilized by any sperm ascending.

'In Britain alone,' Mr Gwillim told the students, '2 per cent of all female adults have blocked tubes. To be sure if these tubes could be opened or reconstructed through surgery many women so afflicted would no longer be infertile.'

Surgery, even in those pre-war days when I was a medical student, could help a small minority of women with occluded tubes. But the vast majority were less fortunate and had their long-held hopes of having a family thwarted irrevocably. And so it remains to this day, despite the advances in surgical techniques. Too often gynaecologists like Mr Gwillim, before and since the war, have had to be truthful and tell the dismayed patient, 'I'm afraid you will never . . . .' *Never.* That verdict of 'never', though softly-spoken, leaves the woman shaking, empty, her face too naked, her private grief too unconcealed. That word 'never' is one I have heard enunciated in gynaecological Outpatients and wards too often over the years. I have had to say it myself. Many times.

But now Mr Gwillim was telling us, 'I would remind you that, when a woman who has been married for a number of years, asks why it is she cannot have a baby there are other causes besides tubal occlusion and the fault, if fault it can be called, is not always to be found in the female partner. In at least one-third of cases the male is solely responsible. In this particular case though . . . .' Mr Gwillim hesitated and turned to a nurse. 'Ask the patient to step in, please.'

I can't remember the name of that patient whose case-history I had recorded in St George's Hospital and who soon appeared through the door. But I recall how she had asked me earlier, 'What have I done wrong?' and how facing Mr Gwillim intensely, quietly, she said, 'I want a baby, doctor, I want one of my own.' I was a student and I felt for her deeply. There have been so many other women since then expressing the same longings, the same unnecessary guilt feelings, and I, older, a gynaecologist myself, have felt the same rush of sympathy for them.

Mr Gwillim spoke to her with great tact and delicacy but she looked uncomprehendingly towards her own X rays on the lit screen, and the students, I among them, shifted uneasily.

The consultant explained how her Fallopian tubes were severely distorted and blocked as a result of some previous infection but it became evident that the patient did not understand what was meant by Fallopian tubes. So Mr Gwillim began at the beginning, explaining everything gently.

'When a female egg-cell, an ovum, is released by a woman's ovary it may proceed into those tubes that lead into and are attached to the womb – the Fallopian tubes. Then, after sexual intercourse, one of the many sperms swimming up from the opposite direction, may meet that egg, may enter it and, as they say, fertilize it. That's the beginning of pregnancy, that's how the baby begins. For the fertilized egg soon divides into two cells, into four cells, and so on, becoming bigger and burrowing into the nourishing wall of the mother's womb. There it develops for nine months until the baby is ready to be born . . . . But if the egg can't descend down the Fallopian tubes because these are obstructed in the first place, none of that can happen.'

The patient then asked an astonishing question. 'Doctor, can't the Fallopian tubes which you say are blocked be by-passed?'

'Oh no,' Mr Gwillim said, looking at the students. We shook our heads.

We knew that if the Fallopian tubes could not be reopened or reconstructed satisfactorily there was no way the sperm could reach the egg to fertilize it. The egg could not be taken from a woman's ovary, placed in a laboratory culture dish and her husband's sperm added to fertilize it. Nor could such a hypothetical fertilized egg be then placed into the same woman's womb to burrow into its wall, to be nourished there, to develop, to grow, to become, after nine months, a normal, much-desired and much-to-be-loved baby. No, we students did not think of such possibilities in those pre-war days.

So no hope was given to the patient that afternoon in the Outpatients at St George's. Mr Gwillim had to say, 'I'm so sorry.' The patient had to leave the hospital defeated; later that evening I thought of her plight as I played the piano at my digs, played perhaps a Beethoven or Schubert sonata, as was my wont when I found myself in certain moods and is still my habit today. I did not know of course – in those days before the war – that one day the quest of by-passing the blocked Fallopian tubes would be one I would share with a Dr Bob Edwards.

Round about the time that same patient had to leave St George's Hospital without hope, a Harvard scientist, Dr John Rock, thought that he had actually managed to fertilize a human egg *in vitro* – that is, in the laboratory, outside the body (literally translated 'in glass'). He reported that he had seen this fertilized egg divide into three cells. His claims were discounted. Dr John Rock's observation of the three cells was considered by other scientists to be merely an example of parthenogenesis – that is to say, the egg had been stimulated to divide without being fertilized by a sperm. In subsequent years similar claims by others were also shown to be mistaken.

Thus when Bob Edwards and I eventually made our quest public, scientists still did not truly believe that laboratory fertilization of the human egg was feasible. Many, if they considered the matter at all, thought such a procedure undesirable: the notion of initiating human life *in vitro* being repugnant to them, unacceptable in principle. Some were fearful of the physical consequences of fertilization *in vitro*. They asked, 'Supposing the baby born is abnormal, a cyclops say, or some other monster?' One American Protestant theologian, Paul Ramsey of Princeton, even declared that he half-hoped that the first child born through such a method would be impaired and be publicly displayed!

Though our aspirations were only to help women like that patient who years ago in Outpatients had whispered to me, a mere medical student, 'What have I done wrong not to have a family of my own?' we certainly had to face opposition – sometimes from colleagues in the medical and scientific world on both sides of the Atlantic. So throughout our work, throughout our collaboration, we have had to be alive to the ethical considerations that are a natural accompaniment of the trend of scientific

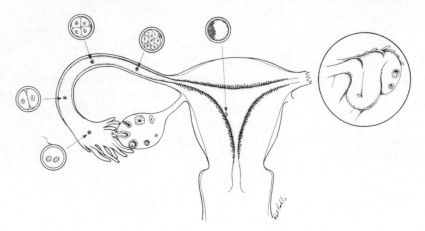

An ovum released by a woman's ovary may proceed into the Fallopian tubes. One of the many sperms swimming in the opposite direction may meet the egg and fertilize it. The fertilized egg divides into two cells, four cells and so on (as shown in the small additional drawings) before burrowing into the wall of the mother's womb. The Fallopian tubes may become distorted and blocked (inset right) preventing the fertilization of the egg by the sperm.

research and medical practice we undertook. We have had to confront objections raised and to resolve genuine doubts expressed. Most of the time though our preoccupations have not been concerned with ethics; rather they have been dense with scientific speculations, technical problems. For on the way to our goal we experienced many setbacks, many disappointments, numerous difficulties.

The collaboration between Bob, a scientist trained in genetics, embryology and immunology, and myself, a doctor specializing in gynaecology, endures in confidence and friendship. Our collaboration began when we met each other in 1968. The quest began even before our meeting – more than a decade earlier when Bob observed fertilized mouse eggs while a very young scientist working in a laboratory in Edinburgh. The quest reached its culmination when both of us heard one Tuesday night in July 1978 – we shall never forget it – the longed-for, normal cry of a baby, conceived out of the womb and now born in an operating theatre in the Lancashire town of Oldham where for many years I have worked and near which I have long lived. The delighted mother of that baby was a young woman not too different, I dare say, from many other childless women I have seen over the years, desperate that they should not remain irrevocably barren – indeed not utterly different from that patient who once attended Mr Gwillim's Outpatients at St George's Hospital and who walked out into the streets of pre-war London tearful and without hope.

2
The Second Chance
Robert Edwards

It was my last year in the University at Bangor in North Wales and I realized that I had made a mistake. Demobbed two years earlier from the Army, I had elected to study agriculture. Now, in 1951, I had decided that I was not particularly interested in seeds of wheat, seeds of oats or seeds of barley – certainly not in how many of them needed to be sown, for efficiency's sake, into any one acre of land. I was on the wrong road and it was a costly error. Being an ex-serviceman, I was considerably older than those students who had not been conscripted to do their National Service and who had come to university straight from school. Worried, I switched to the Department of Zoology. At least I would be more intrigued by animal seeds – by ova, by spermatozoa.

I had long been interested in the scientific processes of reproduction. While a schoolboy, because of gunfire, the bombs falling and the searchlights fumbling the night skies of Manchester, I had been evacuated. I had spent one year on an isolated hill farm in the Yorkshire Dales; there, in the natural laboratory behind hedgerows, wooden gates, byre and barn doors, I had watched with wonder the birth of calves, sheep, pigs, foals, as the aeroplanes of war droned on a long way overhead. During those wartime days I asked myself schoolboy questions about fertilization and birth. Now, in the Department of Zoology, I asked more complicated questions as I attended tutorials or lectures on fertilization and on the early stages of animal life – that is to say, on embryology. On one occasion in the Zoology lab I looked up from a microscope thinking: *Why does only one spermatozoon enter an egg?*

'A million million spermatozoa,' wrote Aldous Huxley, 'all of them alive,' and he continued amusingly:

Out of this cataclysm but one poor Noah
Dare hope to survive.
And among that billion minus one
Might have chanced to be
Shakespeare, another Newton, a new Donne –
But that One was Me.

When the summer examinations arrived, the One that was Me
did not do well. I had changed direction too late. All I managed
to obtain was an ordinary degree without honours.

I was disconsolate. It was a disaster. My grants were spent and
I was in debt. Unlike some students I had no rich parents who
could bail me out. In the Army I had been given a commission
and the Officers' Mess had disclosed to me another world – one
of affluence and grace. There had been croquet on a green lawn.
This had hardly been my style. I was the competitive second son
of a working-class family. My playground had been the rough
streets and back-lanes first of Batley, a small Yorkshire town, and
then of Manchester where, with my brothers and parents, I had
lived in a succession of crowded, argument-laden rented rooms.
I could not write home, 'Dear Dad, please send me £100 as I did
badly in the exams. I owe people and I'm broke.' I had been in
the Army, I had been a student for three years. I was 26 and
skint and finished in Bangor, not knowing quite where to turn
next.

One of my friends was John Slee. One afternoon as we walked
to the tennis courts he told me how he had decided to take a
postgraduate course in genetics at Edinburgh University.
Genetics interested me too – it had been part of the Zoology
course. I had not realized it existed as a separate subject. John
Slee explained that the Professor of Animal Genetics at Edinburgh was the noted embryologist and geneticist Conrad Hal
Waddington. I thought for a glum moment how, alas, my
ordinary degree would in no way commend me to someone like
Waddington. And yet, why shouldn't I have a go? Why shouldn't
I send a letter off to Professor Waddington? What had I to lose?

The envelope addressed to Professor C. H. Waddington, Institute of Animal Genetics, West Mains Road, Edinburgh 9, was in
my handwriting. I dropped it into the pillar box. I did not expect
a favourable reply. I was the clever, ambitious, scholarship boy
who looked as if he had now fallen flat on his face. I expected no
reprieve. Imagine my pleasure then, my sense of relief, when I

was accepted at the Institute.

Now I had to solve the problem of penury. Working one's way through college is not an English tradition. But I had no choice. At once I sought a job. I continued that summer to accept any job, anywhere, however brief. I laboured all day and half the night at hay-time in Yorkshire, journeyed to Wiltshire for the harvest. I carried bananas in Manchester Docks, I took a menial job in a newspaper office, I heaved sacks in a flour mill. I did this until I had accumulated enough cash to pay for my tuition fees and books and for the cost of three months' lodging in Edinburgh. In addition, as an ex-officer, I approached the Officers' Association for £50.

In October, along with ten other students, I was installed in a large Edinburgh, greystone house in Blantyre Terrace, Brunts-field. John Slee had found digs round the corner. I had the overwhelming feeling that I was a lucky man.

Autumn comes early to Edinburgh. In the evenings, when sudden lights in lofty freestone houses and in elegant shops paradoxically darken the city, the wind rises cold and fierce. It hustles the rusting leaves of the public gardens adjacent to Princes Street towards a premature oblivion. But I liked Edinburgh in October. I came to like it in every season, even when those chilling sea-mists crept in from the north. More importantly, I liked the work I was doing. At least I faced the right direction and I gained a more detailed understanding of genetic inherit-ance, embryology, animal breeding, evolution and the amazing growth of cells. 'A man's character is his destiny,' wrote the Greek philosopher Heraclitus, 2500 years ago. To a large degree, a man's character is determined by his genes, and though I did not know it for certain then my own destiny was being deter-mined in that Institute of Animal Genetics.

While learning much from Waddington's approach, as I stud-ied the embryology of flies and frogs, I cast envious eyes at other students who were privileged to work in the Institute under the leading mouse geneticist, Douglas Falconer. For, above all, I wanted to study the reproductive cells of mammals. In my second term – after a spell earning more money by baking bread during the Christmas vacation – I did have some opportunity to study the embryology of mice. This delighted me. Not that mice on first, or even on second, acquaintance are the most attractive of mammals. I can understand and sympathize with those protected ladies who, confronted with one single specimen, tend to run for cover or jump on a table.

I also had to force myself to come to terms with the habits of these vermin – with their pervasive musty smell, their squealings and scrabblings, their ugly new-born progeny which without their fur are nakedly red, their nasty proclivity to bite one's fingers as they are picked up by tail and by scruff of neck. Rats, in comparison, are much more attractive. Lab rats become friendly, they will greet the scientists working with them, and indeed some technicians become so attached to them they take them home. But those quick, agile mice are altogether less lovable. Yet come to terms with them I did, we all did – for mice offer great scope to embryologists and geneticists. Their rapid rate of reproduction enables large numbers of them to be handled and classified with ease. And though my hands, with each month that passed, were bitten more and more by those bad-tempered mice I became increasingly interested in their habits and in their embryos.

I had been fortunate that Professor Waddington had accepted me at the Institute. Now, towards the end of the academic year, he did me another great kindness. Evidently pleased with the work I was doing, he promised to take me on as a Ph.D. student if my examination results were good enough. What an incentive for me to work even harder. I had messed up my student days in Bangor but now I was allowed another opportunity, a chance to embark on real scientific research – to become a real scientist. Of course it would take three more years to complete a doctorate. I would be broke for at least another three years. On the other hand, Professor Waddington did hint strongly that a small amount of money might be found from the University of Edinburgh to support me during my research project.

Those months after Easter were decisive for me. Not only did I study strenuously for the exams but also I keenly attended seminars given by different staff members of the Institute. For all the time while listening to them I was pondering on what research I would undertake if, as now seemed possible, I should stay on at Edinburgh to do a Ph.D.

One afternoon I went to a lecture by Alan Beatty, who was an expert on fertilization and the development of embryos in mice. He had recently made a film called 'Inovulation' with the Film Unit of the Institute. In it he showed how a fertilized mouse egg had been taken from the uterus (womb) of one mouse and injected into the uterus of another mouse. The fertilized egg had subsequently grown into a foetus and then into a healthy new-born mouse. The point about Alan Beatty's work was that the fertilized egg had been transferred into the recipient womb *via the cervix* – the same route whereby artificial insemination is effected. Nobody had successfully transplanted mouse eggs in this way before.

As I sat with John Slee at the back, listening to this dark-haired man in his mid thirties, whose face was full of mobile expression and who was inclined to laugh out loud, I became more and more excited. He was discussing methods whereby chromosomes of a mouse embryo could be modified. There and then I knew what I wanted to do as a Ph.D. student and who I wanted to supervise me. So, as soon as Alan Beatty's lecture was over, I approached him and he nodded, saying, 'Yes, providing your examination results are satisfactory.' They were satisfactory. Professor Waddington was as good as his word. The University of Edinburgh offered me £240 per annum for three years. Hardly a princely sum, but I could not have been more content if I had won the football pools. For at last I had the chance to plan my own research, to read about my chosen topic in detail, to follow the tenuous, exciting leads of my predecessors who sometimes had worked years before, decades before, even centuries earlier. They too had been interested in fathoming the secrets of fertilization and in delving into the mysteries of the newly formed and developing embryo.

3
The Mouse House
Robert Edwards

My supervisor, Alan Beatty, had succeeded in modifying the number of chromosomes in mouse embryos by exposing fertilized eggs to a variety of stimuli. Mice usually have forty chromosomes in their cells, a set of twenty from each parent, and these contain the genes deciding all of the inherited characteristics of the embryo. As a result of Alan Beatty's modifications, some of his embryos lacked a complete set of chromosomes – scientists call them haploid embryos. Others had one or even two extra sets, and so had sixty or eighty in their cells; these were called triploid and tetraploid embryos. This manipulation of embryo cells is a form of genetic engineering, and because of its potential application to domestic animals it could be a valuable tool in agriculture. It involves the manipulation of eggs at fertilization, and my own efforts were to be my first modest introduction to genetic engineering in animals.

It is a long way from mice to men in this respect. Even so, it gave me a valuable foretaste of later debates about human eggs. Any form of genetic engineering in man must raise many eyebrows. There are those who object and pose questions about the ethical propriety of any such manipulations because they own, as I hope I do, a moral sensibility. Others are exercised because their imaginations have already been dramatically doom-lit and gaudily coloured by science-fiction fantasies and visions – fantasies of horror and disaster, and visions of white-coated, heartless men, breeding and rearing embryos in the laboratory to bring forth Frankenstein genetic monsters.

I shall, later, discuss my views about such matters. For the present let me say, simply, that in electing to work under Alan Beatty I had decided to develop new methods to modify the chromosomes of mouse embryos and I had no moral qualms about such investigations. I expected, of course, to learn much, to contribute a little to the pool of general scientific knowledge, and eventually to be rewarded with a Ph.D. I also hoped, albeit vaguely at this juncture, that somehow my work would lead somewhere – perhaps down a pathway that ultimately would be of practical help to mankind.

My first project took me over to Douglas Falconer's Mouse House. This low, ramshackle building, well equipped for scientific research, was conveniently situated at the rear of the Institute. The research I was to do at this paradise of mousery with its mouse inhabitants of all varieties, all shapes and bizarre forms, may seem to be a long way from my later work on human embryos – yet without the knowledge I was to gain in Edinburgh my later discoveries would not have been possible. So here it all began as I confronted large mice, small mice, fat mice, lean mice, mice with curly moustachios and droopy ears, mice that waltzed or simply jerked their way through their mouse-life in the service of genetic research. They were fed and watered, cleaned and dusted, and all their cares met by a bevy of charming Scottish girls. Master of this Hilton Hotel for mice was the benevolent Douglas Falconer. And as I strode along between the cages, five tiers high, I would encounter occasionally other Ph.D students, many of whom had come from Greece, from Egypt, from all over the world to this Mouse House, with eager intentions of seeking new knowledge and wisdom, and as determined as I was to make the most out of these peculiar hotel guests, these myriad rodents.

Alan Beatty agreed that my initial efforts should be directed towards making haploid embryos. By inactivating the chromosomes in spermatozoa I would prevent them from contributing to the embryo. This work involved manipulation of spermatozoa, eggs or embryos and it turned out to be a very trying business. Hundreds of mouse embryos can result merely by pairing male and female mice and leaving the rest to nature. Conception is quite a different and more difficult story – as it is in all mammals – when the spermatozoa must be collected, treated in order to alter their chromosome constitution, then used for fertilization at the critical moment of ovulation.

Female mice had to be identified when in oestrus, that is to say during that period of potential mating and ovulation. Only then could the eggs be fertilized. So these little rodents demanded more and more of my attention.

I hardly had time now to meet John Slee or my new Greek friend Pantelouris, who had been on the same diploma course. Even dates with girl-friends ceased to be frequent because of the demands of the mice. One reason for this was because mice become most active and mate at the dead of night. So their habits turned my project into a succession of night shifts. A stranger that autumn and all that winter, walking after midnight behind the Institute of Animal Genetics, would have observed the lights burning in Douglas Falconer's low-slung Mouse House, and if he had knocked and come in he would have discovered me classifying dozens of female mice or collecting spermatozoa from the males to perform solemnly the act of artificial insemination.

That was a difficult enough task in itself without the genetic engineering, the more experimental side. So when, after four months in the Mouse House, Alan Beatty asked me how I was getting on I could only reply forlornly, 'Two! All I've managed to produce is just *two* embryos.' Alan was suitably sympathetic and encouraging. I returned to my night shifts with renewed vigour.

Perhaps it was this late-night solitary work that led me to wonder more acutely than ever about Life with a capital L. Suddenly I began to read much philosophy. Professor Waddington encouraged us to broaden our interests and his science library was full of books on philosophy and art which were available to any student. He sometimes held debates with theologians and others, and these were very intriguing and enjoyable.

My religious background had hardly been fervent. True, as a boy I had been pushed off to Sunday school in the usual way, but now I began to attend experimentally the different churches in Edinburgh. I tried them all – the Presbyterian, the Episcopal, the Free Church of Scotland, the Methodist, the Baptist, the Congregational, the Lutheran, the Catholic, the Plymouth Brethren, the Quakers. I lingered in churches with stained-glass windows and in those which boasted only plain glass. I looked up at hammer-beam roofs, at those with medieval vaulting and those with plain ceilings. I knelt down between walls that were decorated with murals and those that were blank and devoid of any decoration. Some buildings were dark and seemingly spiritual; others, more rooted in the bustling material life of Edinburgh, appeared more like meeting places. I suppose – looking back on it now – I can say I was on a church crawl: I must have been searching for something. However, I did not become God-intoxicated. I felt eventually that the numinous and the myste-rious could be found rather in the laboratory where each night I peered through a microscope at primitive sex cells. Truth to tell, I found scientific concepts more to my taste than theological fumblings.

My night work gradually began to pay off. I became more proficient. It wasn't until the summer, though, that my methods so improved that I was able to produce a steady trickle of embryos. Not until then could I really turn to the experimental side of the equation. Before the end of the year my success at artificial insemination – still working at dead of night – began to rival the fornicating efforts of the mice themselves. At last I could expose spermatozoa to X rays, to ultraviolet light, and to a variety of drugs, to discover whether I could inactivate their chromosomes. I was now privileged to examine dozens upon dozens of embryos in their earliest stages of growth – and my horizons in research expanded. That winter of 1953, I met my future wife, Ruth Fowler, who had been trained in genetics with a distinct physiological basis. She, too, had elected to do her Ph.D on some of Douglas Falconer's mice but hers had been especially selected for their size: very large giant mice, or very small dwarf mice – both small and large being evidence of the extraordinary skill of the geneticist. I'm afraid at this point I shall have to disappoint the romantic reader, for Ruth and I did not, as they say, 'fall in love at first sight'. I was involved with another girl and Ruth too had a boy-friend. Even when, after a lecture of a statistical nature, we exchanged notes on statistics I did not particularly notice hers!   At Christmas, I returned home to Manchester, feeling certain now that I was more than half way over the hill with regard to my Ph.D work. As usual I went home by bus – for though it took twice as long as the train to reach Manchester from Edinburgh it was but half the price. I was still very short indeed of cash. On the bus, a very, very pregnant lady sat next to me. She worried me a great deal. I felt certain she would go into labour before we reached our destina-tion. If so, what would I do! I was more accustomed to pregnant mice than pregnant women.

At home, I was fussed over as usual by my mother. She felt Edinburgh in winter must be like the North Pole. But I agreed with that Scotsman who averred that Edinburgh could produce great men because the climate was cold enough to stimulate the brain but not so icy as to sap all the imaginative powers of a man in working out how to keep warm. For my part, I was looking forward to my return to the so-called Athens of the north to pursue the work which would lead to my thesis on changing chromosomes in mice embryos.

For the next year the mice proved faithful allies as I counted and classified their chromosomes and they gave me the haploids I required. Most of them were highly abortive in their growth. I also managed to develop simple methods for producing triploids and tetraploids. These developed a little better for three or four days. My experiments proved helpful in later years for human embryos were found to have similar problems which are the cause of many abortions.

One night I decided to leave the mice to their own devices, since I had asked Ruth to come with me to a concert. Afterwards, over coffee, I sucked at an empty pipe and I told her something of my background. Of the fraternal arguments I had had in our early council house in Manchester – how we three young boys all had had a competitive spirit – how we were all determined to win or, if not to win, at least to go down fighting – and how I, now 28, was still determined to succeed.

Ruth looked at me sympathetically with her candid blue eyes and I felt encouraged to tell her how, when I was 11, my mother had altered the direction of my life. I had been offered a place in the Manchester Central High School and she had *insisted* that I accepted.

'When I was at school,' I told Ruth, 'I admired four men particularly. Four scientists – Rutherford, Mendel, Mendeleev and Luke Howard.'

These men, in fact, were still my models: Rutherford, who had at one time taught in Manchester and who formulated the theory that the atom is not indivisible but consists of a nucleus around which electrons revolve in planetary orbits; Mendel, the Austrian monk who experimented with peas and who demonstrated that the characters of parents of cross-bred offspring reappear in certain proportions in successive generations and according to particular laws; Mendeleev, the Russian chemist, who was especially noted for his researches in the subject of the Periodic Law; and Luke Howard, who was the first man to classify the clouds in the sky – cirrus, stratus, cumulus and nimbus.

Ruth was smiling at me faintly. Perhaps I had been a bit pompous. I took the pipe out of my mouth. 'I'm the grand-daughter of Rutherford,' she said, shattering me. 'And curiously, Luke Howard was also an ancestor of mine.' 'You're joking,' I said. She was not joking. *The same genes as Rutherford,* I thought, *my God!* I knew she was from Cambridge but I had not realized she had such a different background from mine. I lit my pipe and did not say much more. Soon I took her home. I did not date her again for months. How could anyone make a pass at a relation of Luke Howard, at a grand-daughter of Rutherford!

Better to return to my night duties with the mice, I thought, and be undistracted. And so I did. I worked night after night, week in, week out, month by month until I had accumulated enough data to enable me to begin my thesis. It took me a long time to write – six months – but the examiners passed it without my being required to submit to an oral examination. When, that July, I played tennis again with John Slee and he served me, as was his habit, another ace, this time he called out, 'Forty – love, *Dr* Edwards.'

4
Night into Day

Robert Edwards

I had so many ideas I wanted to follow up. With my doctorate out of the way I could embark on new studies with other research scientists at the Institute who could provide me with their own expertise. I was not tired of working with mice. I was, though, 'browned off' with having to work continual night shifts, especially as I was beginning to see Ruth Fowler again. If only the mice could be induced to become more sexually active during the civilized hours of nine to five!

Mice could not be given some magic aphrodisiac – horn of rhinoceros, bones of a fairy. On the other hand, perhaps a mouse-night could be turned into a mouse-day. Had not Alan Gates – a young American researcher at the Institute – and Alan Beatty been stimulating the ovaries of immature mice with gonadotrophins? These hormones induced oestrus and ovulation, and perhaps the ovaries of adult mice could be persuaded to ripen their eggs during the office hours. That would be marvellously convenient. Yes, I would approach Alan Gates about it sometime.

Meanwhile, late one night while I was working in the Mouse House, the door opened suddenly to disclose a young post-doctoral worker from Argentina. His name was Julio Sirlin. He had just come off the plane and yet, vibrating with energy, seemed ready to start work at once. I asked Julio to remove the lid from a particular cage. In the blink of an eyelid six furry dwarf mice jumped a yard into the air, momentarily startling him, and making me laugh. It was a favourite pastime of us all in the Mouse House to persuade unsuspecting visitors to remove the lid from the cage of the dwarf mice. They leaped up so high their little bodies seemed as light as helium. Now the six diminutive creatures disappeared in all directions over the floor. It took us half an hour on hands and knees to recapture them.

Julio Sirlin became a great friend of mine. Soon we were sharing a three-roomed flat in Spottiswoode Road, Marchmont, and, of course, I introduced Ruth to him. We also began to collaborate scientifically. He was skilled in the biochemistry of development and in the art of radioactive tracers. He and I managed to produce radioactive mouse spermatozoa which hardly did the mice much good but told us a great deal about their testes. We built tracers into embryos and looked at the synthesis of proteins and nucleic acids in a manner which was novel at the time. Julio was the first man with whom I collaborated who was prepared to work at my pace.

Profitable as our research was, we only gained success by stubbornly marching into the Mouse House when everybody else was going home or pushing off to the pub or to a party or cinema. At least it saved me from spending money. I was still short of cash – especially as Julio was a huge meat-eater so that our conjoint budget for food increased alarmingly as he devoured Argentinian-sized steaks. I was partly to blame too, for I had developed a taste for different clarets. But by December, when Ruth and I became officially engaged, I felt even more keenly that it was absurd working night after night.

I approached Alan Gates who agreed to add his expertise to mine. Alan was five feet six or thereabouts in height, short-haired, correct, meticulous, and polite as are so many academic East Coast Americans. He had carried out impeccable hormone research for many years. His gonadotrophic hormone preparations sounded like a recipe for a witch's brew: take serum from a pregnant mare – this contained gonadotrophins – and inject it into an immature mouse; follow this up two days later with a drop of serum from a pregnant woman – more appropriate hormones in this human serum – and almost unbelievably vast numbers of eggs, not just a few, would hurry to ripen in the ovary, sometimes as many as one hundred! If these immature mice with their over-laden ovaries were allowed to mate with a full-blooded male, then dozens of embryos would be for the taking – and not necessarily at night.

It amazed me to see how casually Alan produced so many dozens of embryos through these activating hormones. Why, for years, I had struggled to obtain just two or three from each mouse. It was ironic. Yet there was a snag. These immature mice had wombs that were too small to nourish crowds of embryos.

They all died after three or four days. The only thing he could do was to transplant the little embryos into a recipient mature mother-mouse whose womb was big enough to sustain their growth. This transplantation operation was very tricky to do. 'If only the hormones worked on *mature* female mice in the first place,' I sighed.

But it was well-known that gonadotrophic hormones did not affect the mature ovary of the mouse or indeed of other mammals. Ruth, too, was interested in hormones, especially those that made mice big or small, for she had elected to do her Ph.D in the genetics of body size. We had talked about our respective research projects over cups of coffee in the Common Room in the Institute, between the cages in the Mouse House, at her apartment (which she shared with three other girls) and in our top attic flat in Spottiswoode Road. Now, as we walked together between those four-storey Edwardian tenements, I suggested that we should work together – on the reproductive hormones of the giant and the dwarf mice.

We did. First we examined these different-sized mice in order to analyse their fertility. We counted their eggs, examined their spermatozoa, investigated their mating behaviour, studied their successful and unsuccessful pregnancies. The small mice would rarely mate and some of the giant mice, too, were so fat and lazy they appeared loth to couple with each other. It seemed the small rodents were like Peter Pan mice – they did not grow up. So, not being truly adult, being immature, presumably they would respond to injections of Alan Gates's hormones? We injected them. As an afterthought, we gave the giant mature mice the same treatment. It was worth a try – the unexpected could always occur, despite scientific and medical dogma insisting that the ovaries of adult females would not respond to gonadotrophic hormones being, since puberty, set irrevocably in their ways.

After the hormone injections, we placed the large and small mice with active males and waited to see what would happen. Most of the small mice mated and ovulated. Surprisingly, so did many of the big mice. Moreover, a few autopsies revealed far more eggs than we believed possible – not only in the Peter Pan mice but in the mature large females as well! When we peered through a microscope at the eggs we discovered they had been fertilized irrespective of the size of the female. We were startled. What a bonus!

We told Alan Gates. He looked dubious. 'Are you sure?' he asked.

We told John Slee. He laughed.

We told Alan Beatty. He was puzzled. 'You'd better check,' he said. We were confident. We had proved that scientific dogma regarding hormones and the mature ovary was hopelessly wrong. Of course we would repeat the experiment, but now we wondered what would happen to those multiple embryos. They were only in their very early stages and naturally the mice did not look pregnant. Would the embryos keep growing? Surely they would degenerate? We decided to leave the Mouse House for a couple of weeks, delighted so far with what had happened.

Most of the next two weeks we spent in the Lake District, enjoying the natural beauty of the scenery, the tons of fresh air, the walks and climbs hand in hand. We did not always talk about hormones and fertilization and mice.

'We can't get married,' I said, leaning over a lichened stone bridge, 'till we save enough money.'

Ruth shook her head. We both looked down at the clear water bubbling along below us. 'That's silly,' she said. She suggested that I should save £125, then we could think about it concretely. 'Then we'll spend that £125 on a honeymoon,' insisted Ruth.

Returned to Edinburgh, we went straight to the cages of the pregnant mice. Large mice, average mice, small mice – it was unbelievable – were all visibly pregnant. More than that, they were superbly pregnant, superlatively pregnant. Excited, we autopsied some of them immediately. There were foetuses everywhere. Gently we withdrew the uterus from the mass of intestines, kidneys and other organs. Foetuses appeared from behind the liver, foetuses adjacent to the kidneys, foetuses tucked between the folds of the alimentary canal. One female carried thirty-seven baby mice, living and perfectly normal.

'Come and look at this,' called Ruth. Our colleagues were looking over our shoulders. Of course, not all the foetuses were alive – in overcrowded wombs some foetuses had died and degenerated. Of these only the small, decaying placenta were visible. But indisputably the mice had mated, ovulated, carried astonishing armies of embryos almost to birth, and the majority had survived despite overwhelming odds – the body weight of the mothers was actually less than the combined weights of their foetuses. And yet orthodox scientific opinion held that the mature ovary was not susceptible to gonadotrophic hormones! Our colleagues nodded, left us to it, went back to continue their own work.

Importantly, most, if not all, of these eggs that we had artificially induced to ovulate were clearly normal; they had been fertilized, they were capable of sustained development. Perhaps we had not merely discovered a means of obtaining as many eggs as any research scientists may require – not just ovulation to order, foetuses when needed, night or day – but there were other exciting prospects: what about affecting super ovulation in farm animals? How valuable that might be! And what about human beings? Those women who had difficulty in having children – could not they be helped?

We had no experimental facilities to go forward in this direction. This was the Mouse House. All we could do was to repeat our work painstakingly, using different strains of mice, testing different hormone injections, counting the eggs, checking fertilization, measuring embryonic deaths, recording the number of live births, looking for anomalies, and generally tying up the whole thing. We had to search the Mouse House for every spare female rodent. Those Scottish girls were terrific, providing us with cage after cage of their assorted stock. There was no doubt about our results. Every strain of mouse responded similarly. They could be made to ovulate by day or by night, four times successfully within a few days, and even to carry litters sired by two males on different days.

'Supposing we put the eggs in a culture fluid, added the hormones, so stimulating them directly, do you think – ?' I began to say to Ruth. But she shook her head. She had her thesis to do. She needed to return to her own work.

It was left to others to carry out similar research on human beings. Some years later, Gemzell in Sweden used substantially the same hormones as we did. What was true for mice was true for women. Hence those multiple pregnancies everybody has read about: twins, triplets, quadruplets, quintuplets, sextuplets. As far as we know Gemzell worked independently of us.

After Ruth had been awarded her Ph.D we settled on a wedding date. I had saved the £125 and we spent it all, every penny of it, as promised, on our September honeymoon in Venice and Dubrovnik. When we returned to Edinburgh I knew it would be our last year there. I wanted to go to the USA – at least

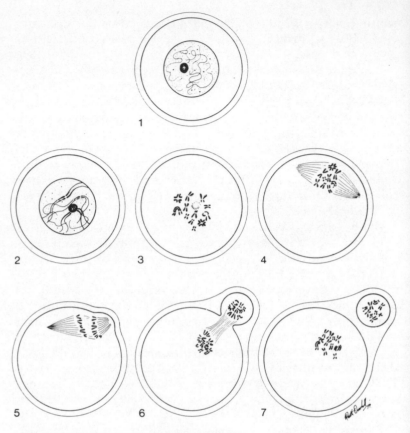

THE MARCH OF THE CHROMOSOMES

'Before the injection each egg in the ovary had the usual large vacuous
nucleus [1] . . . . But two hours after we gave the HCG to the mice an
amazing miniature military-like show began. The large nucleus
gradually disappeared as it condensed into typical chromosomes in the
egg. This was the beginning of the ripening phase [2]. The
chromosomes then moved like soldiers through a prepared drill. First
they marched to the centre of the egg [3], then out to the periphery
[4]. Next they slowly separated into two equal halves as they glided
along a spindle [5]. As if to inaudible military music, one half
marched out of the egg for ever and into a small body known as the
first polar body [6]. The other half remained in the egg [7]. The
purpose of their manoeuvres was to prepare the egg for fertilization
and the precision of it all, as we peered through the microscope, was
breathtaking [facing page].'

for one year. During the war, I had observed the free and easy confidence of American servicemen and later I had heard enthusiastic stories about the USA from many friends. Besides, like so many of my generation, I had seen countless Hollywood films, the skyscrapers and the Open Spaces. Go west, Young Man was to me a glamorous imperative.

But first I was involved in a further discovery in mice. Ruth and I had noticed how the hormones had caused the growing eggs to develop in perfect synchrony. So had Alan Gates with the immature mice. It was like setting accurate alarm clocks. Give the hormone at midday and then at midnight the clamour of bells would all begin together. Indeed, the interval between the second injection, the serum from pregnant women (known professionally as HCG) and ovulation was exactly twelve hours. What happened to the eggs in that twelve-hour interval?

Alan Gates and I decided to find out by examining them under a microscope. We observed unexpected and fascinating changes. Before the injection each egg in the ovary had the usual large vacuous nucleus. It was always like this – one could demonstrate it to the least bright undergraduate. But two hours after we gave the HCG to the mice an amazing miniature military-like show began. The large nucleus gradually disappeared as it condensed into typical chromosomes in the egg. This was the beginning of the ripening phase. The chromosomes then moved like soldiers through a prepared drill. First they marched to the centre of the egg, then out to the periphery. Next they slowly separated into two equal halves as they glided along a spindle. As if to inaudible military music, one half marched out of the egg for ever and into a small body known as the first polar body. The other half remained in the egg. The purpose of their manoeuvres was to prepare the egg for fertilization and the precision of it all, as we peered through the microscope, was breathtaking.

Because of the regularity of these events we could predict all the ripening stages of the mature egg: where the manoeuvres would begin, where the chromosomes would be at a particular time, when the eggs were ready for ovulation and fertilization. Would the timing be the same in farm animals and in human eggs? I wondered, once more thinking of the practical applications of such knowledge. No human ovaries were available at the Institute! Nor, for that matter, were those of farm animals. Again, research along these lines had to be delayed.

And yet now, as I look back at those years in Edinburgh, I am surprised that I left this fascinating area of research to enter new pursuits. It must have been obvious to me that similar things could be done with the eggs of other animals, including man. The pointers were there, indicating the pathway to the earliest stages of human life. Yet off I went in a totally new direction – into immunology. Those meetings I attended at the Institute in which men like Waddington and Beatty discussed wide-ranging possibilities of predetermining the sex of offspring had stimulated me. I felt the precision of immunological methods might help to identify which spermatozoon carried an X female-determining chromosome and which carried a Y male-determining chromosome. I wrote to Albert Tyler, Professor at the California Institute of Technology, for I had read his papers on this very subject. 'The beautiful interaction between sperm and egg resembles the reaction between antigen and antibody,' Tyler had remarked.

I had an affirmative reply from Albert Tyler. Ruth, too, would work on a project on immunology and fertilization. No, we wouldn't be short of money in America especially as the Population Council in New York also had read of the work I had done with Julio on radioactive spermatozoa and awarded me a modest fellowship.

So it was goodbye Edinburgh, though not goodbye Britain, for Alan Parkes, the Head of the Department of Experimental Biology in Mill Hill, London, had told me when he visited Edinburgh, 'Let me know if you ever want a job.' That would be our next stop after California. At one time, in North Wales, everything seemed to have gone wrong and there was no way out. Now, adventures were beckoning us this way and that. We set out cheerfully for the sunshine of California, its unbelievable landscape. We would miss Edinburgh, its stern beauty, the concerts at the Usher Hall, the splendid walks, and of course our friends, our good friends.

Our days and our nights at the Institute of Genetics had been occupied with hard scientific work. We had speculated and argued – but our debates had been essentially innocent of those ethical and social issues that were to engage me so pressingly in my later work. My scientific foundations had been clearly laid in Edinburgh and I was aided, partly by good luck, and partly by the fact that the reproductive cycle of the mouse happens to be a very simple one. It was the end of the Mouse House, its pervasive, musty smell. It was also the end of my years of poverty.

5
The Control Dish
Robert Edwards

It was quite a culture shock to return to drab Britain, to a northern suburb of London, in the autumn of 1958, after having enjoyed one year of fat sunshine in California. People at home were altogether more cautious, almost mean, compared with open-handed Americans. The Americans, living in a consumer society, did not seem to be afflicted with the old British imperative of Save, Save. Their ethic rather was Spend, Spend. But then they had more money. Here we faced Selwyn Lloyd's pay-freeze. There we drove a big beat-up Plymouth that guzzled gas; here we ran a small beat-up Morris 8 that didn't. There we lived in a modern apartment among spacious acres of land; here we had to find temporary digs in a clenched house too full of furniture. There we drove along straight generous roads that went on for ever through desert and below sparse jutting mountains; here we had to change into second gear as we joined slow traffic queues whenever we headed for our beloved Kew Gardens or Hampton Court.

The National Institute for Medical Research at Mill Hill lived up to its name. Everything was geared to research: lavish equipment and facilities, well staffed, plenty of technical assistance, sufficient funds, in fact virtually every facility needed by a young scientist such as myself who was anxious to spread his wings. I intended to continue with my immunology studies: immunology as a possible method of contraception. To vaccinate a woman against becoming pregnant could perhaps become a possibility? The relevance of immunology to animal and human reproduction had always been dubious – there were so many pitfalls, so many half-truths. There were things I wanted to clarify. And I had a five-year contract and was privileged to work with Alan Parkes and the Australian specialist on fertilization in mammals,

Bunny Austin. These were two men whose work I had long admired. (Oddly both of them were to become my Professors in Cambridge in due course.)

When we returned to Britain Ruth was pregnant – we were expecting the baby in January. So with our Californian savings of £1500, I searched for a suitable house in the vicinity of the Institute. Finally, we decided on a freehold property in Deacon's Hill Road in Elstree. The agents wanted £5000. I offered less. Eventually we settled on £4850 and I put down our savings on a mortgage. It was our first house. Soon, in January, we welcomed our first daughter, Caroline.

I enjoyed the Institute and pay my respects to it, but research institutes do tend to be monolithic – there is no let-up from research. In a university there is more variety, there are wider challenges as one teaches undergraduates, encourages Ph.D students and engages in activities which allow one to forget, at least briefly, the knotty problems that befog all research projects at one time or another. I like the glorious swing of the university year – the balance between term-time and vacations. The only sad thing is the current state of university laboratories. Even today in my lab in Cambridge there is not even a piped hot water supply!

But I have digressed. Though immunology continued to be my main preoccupation at Mill Hill, I remained as interested in eggs, in fertilization and genetics as I had been in Edinburgh. I even tried to tame wild hares hoping I might be able to cross them with rabbits. But those hares did not thrive in captivity – they would hardly breed in cages. The Institute was too warm, too comfortable for them! They preferred the frosts of winter outside, the danger not under strip lighting but under the high stars. The hares and rabbits struck back too – as did those thousand ghosts of Edinburgh mice – for gradually I became sensitive to the fur of all these rodents. This allergy persists to this day.

A topsyturvy period of months, even years, ensued. Hamlet at Elsinore might have mused, 'To be or not to be.' I, in Mill Hill, asked myself, 'Immunology or embryology?' For every three weeks that I worked at immunology I worked another on embryology. I flitted from laboratory to laboratory in the UK and the USA, changed scientific and medical partners in a way unmatched in any barn dance. And though I was gaining more than a passable reputation in the immunology of reproduction, the eggs were always there in the background beckoning me on to my real work. I recalled, often, how in Edinburgh I had observed the regularity in the ripening programme of mouse eggs and what had happened when the ovaries had been bombed by those gonadotrophic hormones.

What was decisive in my return to the path of embryology was the sudden explosion of new work done on human chromosomes by numerous scientists and doctors. Human beings, it was now revealed for the first time, should have forty-six chromosomes. The exceptions were children with Down's syndrome (Mongolism) as well as people with some other inherited defects who were shown to have one chromosome too many or too few. The same was true of many foetuses which aborted spontaneously. Some of those aborted foetuses were even more unusual: they were triploids (with sixty-nine chromosomes) or even tetraploids (with ninety-two). No wonder, when I talked over these discoveries with Ruth, we recalled the skittering mice of Edinburgh.

The pace of these discoveries was so rapid, their clinical application so important, that I longed to be involved. But nobody outside a busy hospital could hope to contribute anything. There were no human patients in the Institute and I had to watch from the sidelines. I was firm in the belief that the cause of the great majority of these chromosome upsets arose in the ovary during the ripening programme, when the chromosomes did their amazing manoeuvres and marched like soldiers soon after fertilization. I needed human eggs, though, not mouse eggs, to prove my point.

Our social life continued pleasantly enough. We had new friends and old friends too, such as John Slee, visited us in Elstree. In April 1960, our second daughter, Jennifer, had been born. Our visitors those days would often observe the pram outside in the front garden with its sleeping baby, and Caroline, awake and lively inside, demanding Ruth's attention. One couple whom we liked very much and whom we felt close to, wanted, but could not have, children. When they visited us that autumn and cuddled our babies I could not but be aware of the feelings aroused in them. The trees bore fruit, the clouds carried rain, and our friends, for ever childless, played with our Caroline, our Jennifer.

I think it was their bearable but true predicament along with my preoccupation about ripening eggs and fertilization that made me wonder for the first time about the practicability of replanting human embryos in the womb of a woman. Had I not replanted embryos of mice into the womb of a mouse in Edinburgh myself? Could the jump be made from mouse to man? Perhaps the hormones need not be injected into women but could be added direct to the unripe eggs taken from a human ovary and placed into a culture solution – a solution made up of such ingredients as salt, potassium chloride, glucose, a touch of protein – nourishment for any possible growing embryo. Then HCG directly into that culture dish. Yes. But first I must work again with mice to prove the point. Mice had helped me before. I would try adding HCG directly to mouse eggs in a culture medium.

The experiment proved unbelievably straightforward. Neither the culture fluid nor the hormones presented a problem. Of course, in some dishes, I did not add HCG – I kept these as controls. All was so easy and predictable: vast numbers of mouse eggs went through their programmes like clockwork. Add a spot of HCG to the culture fluid, pop in the eggs and, two hours later, there goes the nucleus and here come the marching chromosomes. I watched it all happening under the microscope with growing excitement. Happily I turned to peer at the control dish, at the eggs to which no hormone had been added. For a moment I held my breath, baffled. Without HCG they should have been unripe, but no – astonishingly *they were ripening too at precisely the same rate and exactly on schedule*. I looked up from the microscope, went to the window and looked down far below into the middle distance at the red rooftops of the suburban houses of London. Perhaps I had made a mistake?

I returned to the microscope. There was no doubt about it. Moreover my experiment, as I discovered, was repeatable. It was all so simple – why, anyone could do it. The eggs taken from the ovary would ripen under their own steam. All they needed was a simple culture medium to go through their whole startling programme just as if the mother had been given HCG. I soon discovered that the eggs of rats and hamsters acted in the same way. Surely the whole field then was in my grasp – cows, sheep, monkeys – and man, too, if I could only get their eggs?

I began to prepare a manuscript announcing my discoveries. First, I had to check the scientific literature to set the background. Upstairs in the Mill Hill Institute there is a very spacious, comprehensive library. I sat there amongst the polished tables

reading the journals hour after hour. One morning, in the quiet
of that comfortable library, as I read one particular paper I
stopped reading and said quietly, 'Sod it.' I looked up. Nobody
had heard me. Nobody in the library at that particular moment
was aware of my sudden disappointment. For I had just learned
that my discovery was not new. The American, Gregory Pincus,
the noted developer of the contraceptive pill, had reported the
same result when he had worked with the eggs of rabbits in a
Cambridge laboratory a quarter of a century earlier. He had
placed them in a culture solution as I had done. He had watched
them ripen in the same way. The programme, he reported, was
an hour or two shorter in rabbits but the method was identical.
But Pincus had gone one step further. He had done the same
thing with human eggs, having removed them from small pieces
of ovary. He described how they followed virtually the same
ripening programme as rabbit eggs. My results were purely
confirmatory – they were not news at all. Pincus had got there
first with rabbits and man.

Research scientists like to be first in their discoveries. I am no
exception. I sat in the Mill Hill Institute library momentarily
depressed; the novelty of my discovery had suddenly worn thin.
It was simply amazing that virtually no one else had followed up
Pincus's work for over twenty-five years. I returned to the
laboratory and told the sad news to my technician-assistant
Gillian Icke, who was just putting on her white coat.

Yet as I drove home to Elstree I pondered, 'Was it so sad?' It
was encouraging in practical terms. Human eggs, according to
Pincus, would ripen outside the body and become ready for
fertilization. That was the real point if I was to be of use one day
to certain childless couples such as our friends. Or if I could find
the cause of Mongolism. I would need to confirm the Pincus
results, of course. Baboons and monkeys were occasionally autopsied at Mill Hill and I would be able to collect their eggs and put
them straight into culture. I would do that. But how to obtain
human eggs – a fresh human ovary or part of one? Such tissue
would have to come from pieces of ovary removed for medical
reasons and I knew no gynaecologist who could help me.

As I parked the car back home in Elstree, Caroline toddled out
to meet me. I picked her up. Caroline had been born at the
nearby Edgware General Hospital. She had been delivered by the
registrar of the consultant gynaecologist, Molly Rose. Perhaps if

I telephoned Molly Rose she would be helpful? I carried Caroline into the kitchen where Ruth was ironing to tell her what I had read in a journal that day at the Institute's library.

6

The Green Chromosomes

Robert Edwards

Molly Rose was a small, vivacious, middle-aged gynaecologist. She went out of her way to help me, making collaboration easy, phoning me without fail before an operation if any possibility arose of a small piece of ovarian tissue becoming available. She introduced me to operating theatre routines, to masks and gowns, to sterile trays, to human beings undergoing surgery.

Dissecting mice and rats, that was one thing. This was utterly different. Here, in the operating theatre, I felt myself to be exactly what I was – a novice. I stood at the back wearing a mask, careful not to touch anything. I obeyed all instructions to the letter. 'Come forward now,' directed Molly and I came forward clutching my glass sterile pot – the receptacle for the precious bit of superfluous ovarian tissue.

Two or three times a month I would be summoned to Edgware General Hospital. I was always immensely impressed by Molly Rose's surgery. And, as I waited for her to call me forward, as I glimpsed the naked skin of another human being being cut and human blood spurting, the clamps applied, I sometimes questioned my right to be there. 'What am I doing?' I asked myself. 'Do I really have a plàce in this theatre?' There, on the operating table, was a woman who had been ill whom Molly hoped to make well again. That was the point, the whole point of those blazing lights, those gleaming instruments, those rapt figures bending over her in the posture of mercy – the surgeon herself, the anaesthetist, the nurses. And I? I was there merely for some spare eggs, for a piece of ovary that had to be removed anyway and which I would take back to my safe laboratory bench in Mill Hill. The eyes swarming above the masks were not unfriendly to me – but the ritual going on here was not academic.

Now that I had a small but regular supply of human ova from

Edgware – and elsewhere, for I had persuaded other gynaecologists to bequeath me ovarian tissue also – I could plan my work. I started with high hopes. After three months I began to feel less certain. Dozens of eggs were cultured. I examined them eagerly after three, six, nine and twelve hours. None of them changed their appearance in any way whatsoever. Their unwinking nuclei gazed back at me steadily whether they had come from rhesus monkeys, baboons or from humans. They would not ripen, their chromosomes marched nowhere at all, no matter which culture medium I used.

After six months my hopes evaporated completely. Pincus, whom I respected and whom I had met two or three times, was wrong, unless somehow he had performed some extra manoeuvre by chance. No, that was not it. Probably primates were too different from rodents, the menstrual and oestrus cycles too different from each other. Yet I decided to try once more, adding this time the old hormone recipe to the culture dish: a drop of blood from a pregnant mare, a peck of HCG. Still nothing moved. After twelve hours those eggs remained stubbornly unchanged.

Pincus had been wrong before. His work on parthogenesis during the 1930s, on the birth of fatherless rabbits, had failed to stand the test of time. All the same, I admired him enormously. Among the famous scientists whom I have met and come to know he still stands near the top. Pincus had helped to reshape modern life, especially for women, with his contraceptive pill. I thought then, as I think now, that he never received full recognition for his work. There are men – pygmies compared with him – who have been awarded Nobel Prizes. Perhaps he was too controversial. Some of his research leading to the Pill, his critical studies, had been carried out not in the USA but in Puerto Rico, where his novel work on patients was perhaps more readily accepted. Despite such questionings I knew him as a man who moved mountains. He was gritty and outspoken. He was a fighter. He would have made a fine Yorkshireman! All the same, as I now discovered myself, his report of twenty-five years ago was, alas, wrong. I was wasting my time.

I decided to return to my studies in immunology. 'At least,' I consoled myself, 'I have become familiar with human eggs, thanks above all to Molly Rose.' Molly had become more than a collaborator. Ruth had become pregnant again and we were delighted. We wanted a third child very much. But at one time the pregnancy was threatened and, worried, we called Molly in for advice. Happily, in November 1962 we had our third baby, a girl again, and Molly Rose delivered her. She was as beautiful as our other two daughters. We called her Sarah.

Sarah, in the Old Testament, after barren years had been blessed late in life and in joy had mothered a child. In any case, because of those close friends of ours, my thoughts often turned to the plight of barren women who seemed irrevocably condemned to childlessness. Yet were they? 'And the angel said .... "Lo, Sarah thy wife shall have a son" .... Now Abraham and Sarah were old and well stricken in age, and it ceased to be with Sarah after the manner of women. Therefore Sarah laughed within herself, saying, "After I am waxed old shall I have pleasure, my lord being old also?" And the Lord said unto Abraham, "Wherefore did Sarah laugh, saying, shall I of a surety bear a child which am old? Is anything too hard for the Lord? At the time appointed I will return unto thee, according to the time of life, and Sarah shall have a son." '

While working on immunology over the next few months, I could not help but dream now and then of eggs. One morning, driving to Mill Hill, it occurred to me that the ripening programme in the eggs of primates might simply take longer than in rodents. Supposing the nucleus changed after twelve hours and only then the chromosomes would become visible? It was just a hunch. But my time at Mill Hill was running out. It was worth a last throw.

It so happened that some rhesus monkeys at the Institute were being autopsied in the late afternoon so I duly collected their ovaries. Soon I was placing a few oocytes in culture. I would examine these eggs at increasing intervals. I returned home to Elstree late that evening. I don't recall what I did that night. There was nothing special about it. No doubt, as usual, I played with my daughters before they went to bed; chatted with Ruth as we ate dinner together; maybe later listened to music or read a book.

Next morning, I looked at one of the eggs under the microscope. Just on twelve hours had passed. As I expected, the unwinking nucleus was still there. I waited three more hours before taking the next egg from the culture and preparing it for microscopic examination. Now fifteen hours had passed, but gazing down on to the illuminated slide I shook my head.

Everything was stationary. I looked at the last egg available after eighteen hours and, suddenly, I felt that old twinge of excitement. Surely the nucleus was beginning to disperse? Yes, yes. Surely the chromosomes were about to appear? But I couldn't be sure. There were no more eggs in the culture left to examine. Damn it. And sadly there were no more monkeys. I left the laboratory frustrated.

I was home at Elstree when Molly Rose called me, saying that there was a possibility of a piece of human tissue becoming available. 'Is it needed?' she asked. I replied with vehemence into the telephone, 'It certainly is.' I drove fast over to the Edgware General Hospital. The following hours were to put me firmly and decisively into the study of human embryology. For I had collected in the operating theatre what I needed. And back at Mill Hill, I placed four valuable oocytes into the culture fluid. All I had to do now was wait, wait. I must not look at them too early. The first one I would examine after eighteen hours. Would I then see what I thought I had seen in the rhesus monkey's egg?

After eighteen hours exactly I looked and saw, alas, the nucleus unchanged – no sign of ripening at all. Failure. Had I made a mistake about the monkey's egg? Impatiently, I looked there and then at a second oocyte. It was like the first. I had to accept that I had drawn a blank. But I had two human oocytes left. I would look at one of them again in six hours' time – by then they would have been in the culture medium for twenty-four hours.

When I next peered down the microscope I could not help but feel elated. Surely something was beginning to move? Just a suggestion, but something. I must be patient. I must not look at the last egg too soon. The next four hours passed slowly, slowly, but when I did examine the final oocyte I felt as much excitement as I had ever experienced in all my life. Excitement beyond belief. At twenty-eight hours the chromosomes were just beginning their march through the centre of the egg. Fine, clear, absolutely visible, a sight to reward all my past efforts. A living, ripening, human egg, unbombarded by any hormones, beginning its programme just as the mouse eggs had done. Now that programme was in its earliest stages, but unmistakably on its predestined way. There, in one egg, in the last of the group, lay the whole secret of the human programme. My hopes of chromosome analysis and of fertilized eggs – the possibility of helping people – had suddenly been brought closer to concrete realization.

I simply had to show the egg to someone else. Under the microscope was a kind of masterpiece and I had to say to someone, 'Come and look.' My nearest colleague, next door, was Mike Ashwood-Smith. We had come to know each other very well indeed in Mill Hill since he arrived to finish his Ph.D and we frequently discussed together our aspirations and doubts. Direct, forthright, ebullient, Mike was working with the ultraviolet microscope at the time, an instrument that makes tissues fluoresce and display all the colours of the rainbow.

At the door of his room, I said, trying to contain my excitement, 'Mike, come and see this egg – it's beginning to work.'

He stood up. 'Are you sure?'

I nodded.

'That's marvellous,' he said, stepping towards me and into my room. When he looked down the microscope he was as delighted as I was. Then with typical bubbling enthusiasm he suggested putting the egg under the ultraviolet microscope. 'Why, we'll get a really beautiful picture of those chromosomes.'

'Hang on,' I said.

After all, I had not photographed the egg or made any record whatsoever. I was far from sure that I wanted Mike messing around. But he was irresistible. He snatched the slide, overruling my misgivings, and took it next door. He added the appropriate stain and put the egg under the ultraviolet microscope. The effect was dynamic.

'Look at that,' said Mike, ecstatically.

I saw lovely green chromosomes shining brilliantly on a yellow background.

'Terrific,' I exclaimed.

'I can do better than that,' said Mike.

I felt another twinge of apprehension. It would be best to photograph it first, to have a record for the future.

'Just one second,' Mike shouted confidently. 'I'll make it better still.'

Even as he spoke he pressed the slide in all directions, trying to make the egg more visible before replacing it under the microscope. When he looked again I realized something was wrong. Mike no longer seemed ebullient. The more he twiddled, looking at the slide, the more clouded his face became. It was my turn to gaze down. No green chromosomes. Nothing at all. We kept looking, we searched for that egg. It had gone. Whatever had been there was obliterated for ever. After an hour we had to give up. Considerably chastened, Mike said, 'Sorry. So sorry.'

It did not matter. True, a record of that egg would have convinced everybody. But what we had seen was no hallucination. It was no dream.

'There'll be other eggs,' I said, smiling at Mike.

He nodded. I returned to my room, thinking what a wonderful sight it had been. Green chromosomes on a yellow background. Why, it meant that possibly infertility in some women could be cured. The angel could come to Sarah. For if the oocyte ripened like that then it might be fertilized *in vitro* – in the test tube, as no doubt some would popularly describe it. There would be those, of course, who would think that such a manoeuvre was wrong, even evil. How could it be so if a barren woman's long suffering could be alleviated?

But there would be problems if I continued thinking along these lines, I knew that. Quite recently I had been to a lecture by Margaret Jackson on artificial insemination of women, given at the Institute. She stood there, five feet nothing, facing all my tall colleagues as they cross-examined her aggressively about the ethical issues insemination raised. But fertilization *in vitro* would arouse even more hostility. Henry James, writing about the art of fiction, held that art lived upon discussion, 'upon experiment, upon curiosity, upon variety of attempt, upon the exchange of views and the comparison of standpoints . . . . Art derives a considerable part of its beneficial exercise from flying in the face of presumptions.' What was good for art was even more true for science.

What I needed now, though, was to expand my work. I scouted around for other sources of ovarian tissue and tried to rally more doctors to my cause – explaining how in Edinburgh I had worked with mice and obtained all those embryos and how it might be possible to obtain similar results in human beings. The response was, perhaps, inevitable. Most interviews followed the same course as I eagerly explained what I needed. 'Inject an infertile woman patient with hormones early in her menstrual cycle, then give a spot of HCG to cause ovulation, perform a small operation twenty-eight hours later and collect her ripening eggs – for that is the time required, as I have seen under the microscope.'

The good doctors began to stare at me dubiously. Manfully, I continued, 'Place the eggs in culture fluid, collect the husband's semen for fertilization *in vitro.*' The doctors were now remembering another appointment and seemed restless. I ploughed on, without much hope of convincing them. I described the growth of embryos in culture and how they could be replaced in the mother's uterus so by-passing, say, any possible blocked Fallopian tubes that had been the cause of infertility.

Perhaps I explained myself badly, or was too enthusiastic. Or the issues of fertilization carried a more emotional charge than I realized. Whatever the cause the door closed behind me and I came away empty-handed. Worse, no further eggs came my way while I was at Mill Hill. Molly did not have any tissue to offer and my other sources also dried up.

What I wanted to do was no secret. Like Margaret Jackson, I was being cross-examined. One day the telephone rang for me. It was a television producer. 'Are you working on human fertilization?' he asked. I tried to explain to him what my problems were.

'How do you propose to achieve fertilization?' he probed.

I could see Alan Parkes who was nearby looking at me, shaking his head negatively, vigorously. He was beginning to write something down on a piece of paper.

'Will you fertilize in a test tube?' asked the TV producer.

'Probably in a Petri dish, a culture dish,' I responded.

'Will you come on a programme on human fertilization?' continued the producer.

'Well,' I began.

Alan Parkes handed me his note. I read, *Don't let yourself be interviewed over the telephone. Take care.*

Others were more aware of the antagonism towards human fertilization than I initially was. And it didn't help when Alan Parkes left for Cambridge. For Audrey Smith, a dynamic, talkative, middle-aged scientist, became the head of my department. She had worked on freezing cells and organs – on freezing sperms too, but she was against human fertilization *in vitro.*

'It is unethical,' she said.

'Why?' I asked.

'Because it is,' she replied.

She must have gone to the retiring Director of the Institute, Sir Charles Harrington, because I was summoned into his office. He rose from his desk and said to me, 'I don't want any human eggs fertilized here.'

In a matter of months Sir Charles had gone. Peter Medawar became Director and had no objection to fertilization. 'Go ahead,' he said. It was too late – at least it was too late at Mill Hill. My five-year stint was coming to an end. But first I read in the library another piece of highly relevant information. It was a paper by M. C. Chang, a widely respected Chinaman who had worked on fertilization for many years in the USA and who had, indeed, collaborated with Pincus in the development of the contraceptive pill. Chang had discovered that the eggs of rabbits, if they ripened entirely in culture, would abort when reimplanted in the womb. It seemed that a *part* of the ripening process had to occur in the ovary before being transferred to the culture dish. That is why he forced the eggs of rabbits to begin ripening first by injecting the does with HCG before letting the ripening process continue in culture. One day I would need to confirm this work, to see whether in humans, too, the eggs would first have to be ripened partly in the body. Now, though, it was time to leave Mill Hill – first for a short spell at Glasgow University, where local gynaecologists helped me to discover that eggs needed something under forty hours to complete their ripening programme and be ready for fertilization, and then in 1963 on to the Physiological Laboratory at Cambridge, to rejoin Alan Parkes.

7
The Road Taken
Robert Edwards

Our new home in Cambridge – 48 Gough Way – a detached house in a brand-new pleasant estate – was spacious enough for a large family. All the same, Ruth was dismayed when she was found to be expecting twins. However large the house, five youngsters sounded like a lot of hard work. 'All those nappies,' she groaned at me. For my part, I was delighted.

The doctor assumed, wrongly, that we would want boys. He nodded knowingly at our three young daughters and quietly said to me, 'Don't worry,' indicating that this time Ruth was sure to have at least one boy. In July, at the hospital, I waited outside the delivery room. When the doctor popped his head around the corner the smile on his face was a little forced.

'It's a girl,' he said. 'Everything's fine.' He hesitated, then cheerily said, 'Don't be anxious – one girl born but there's still one to go.' And he resolutely went back into the delivery room. Soon he was to return looking crestfallen. 'It's another girl,' he said needlessly apologizing. We were happy and excited taking our twins Anna and Meg back home to 48 Gough Way to their three young, elder sisters.

At the Physiological Laboratory, with Alan Parkes once more my head of department, I continued my work on immunology and on the fertilization of eggs. Human eggs were still slow coming my way, despite the fact that I had struck up friendly relations with some of the gynaecologists at Cambridge's Addenbrooke's Hospital. For that reason I worked much more often with the eggs of cows and sheep and monkeys. Perhaps it was no bad thing. I had to clarify the principles underlying the ripening process of the eggs in different species. This would place the human programme in perspective.

Other laboratories donated me a monkey ovary occasionally.

As for ovaries of cows and sheep, these were available by the dozen from the local slaughterhouse. Needless to say, I hardly enjoyed visiting that building in Newmarket Road, despite the kindness of the manager and his staff. It was sad to witness the cows queueing up, to hear the repetitious, peculiarly sharp crack of the gun that stunned each animal, then the soft thud of the creature falling without a cry.

It took me the best part of a year to understand with certainty the ripening programme of the eggs in different species. In all of them the maturation process began quite spontaneously as I had discovered it had in those Edinburgh mice. The eggs of pigs, like those of humans, required a long period to ripen, some thirty-six hours; rodents a few brief hours only; cows and rhesus monkeys an intermediate time. In all species, the programme in my culture appeared to be identical to that occurring naturally in the ovary. So eggs from all these species could be ripened and made ready for fertilization in my culture dishes quite easily.

I was beginning to adapt to the daily Cambridge life. I found certain things hard to take – the all-male, misogynist public-school traditions; the exclusivity of certain Colleges; the privileges given to the already privileged; the absurdity of certain social anachronisms – the students attending formal dinners at their colleges or quaintly wearing gowns when walking the streets of the city or wildly climbing weather-beaten walls after midnight because the gates had been locked. On the other hand, the sheer beauty of the place – the lawns, the bridges over the river, the sunlight shaking beneath them, the weeping willows, all the trees, the boats, the churches, spires, bells – conspired to soothe, console and enchant even a truculent Yorkshireman such as me.

Besides, had not Isaac Newton, Darwin, Rutherford – yes, and Rutherford's son-in-law, Ruth's father, Ralph Fowler, too – all heard these same bells, seen similar eights rowing up to Jesus lock in the early-morning mists? That was part of the Cambridge tradition too – and a Puritan concern with the truth and high seriousness. Whatever antagonisms I nurtured towards snobbishness and nepotism, there was also an ambience of scientific excellence to revere. I was surrounded by so many talented young men and women that I would have been content if only human eggs had come my way more freely.

At that very moment I had three human oocytes ripening in

a culture. I decided to try and fertilize them with my own spermatozoa. I told Ruth my intention. She nodded and said, 'Best of luck.' She knew as well as I did that such an exercise would most probably fail. For, in 1965, it was thought by everybody that spermatozoa had to be exposed to the secretions of the uterus or Fallopian tubes before eggs could be fertilized. Much work had been carried out by scientists of different nationalities and all had concluded that this was the case. For instance, a group of French workers had taken sperms from the uterus of a previously mated doe and had fertilized rabbit eggs with them outside the body – that is in the laboratory. True, Chang – also Yanagimachi, a Japanese working in the USA – had successfully fertilized hamster eggs in culture by using spermatozoa taken directly from the male hamster reproductive tract. Scientists merely assumed hamsters were somehow different, an exception. The dogmatic belief that uterine spermatozoa were needed to fertilize eggs *in vitro* remained unshaken. 'They could be wrong,' I said to Ruth.

So, one evening after dinner, I took out the bicycle and rode down Gough Way towards my little research laboratory where the three eggs in the culture dish were now almost ripe. I had collected them for culture almost thirty-six hours earlier. It was 8 p.m. when I wheeled my bicycle to the Physiological Laboratory. I climbed the four flights of graded stairs and hurried through the winding corridors, past the framed photographs of famous Cambridge scientists on the walls, to my own lab.

Sometimes, at night, I could hear below, across the way, rock music coming from the Regal Cinema or, more distantly, the harmonious sound of a Cambridge University choir. That evening, as I collected my own semen, removed the excess fluid and added my spermatozoa to the eggs in the culture fluid, there was no music or noise at all. Just a tap dripping into the sink. I would examine the eggs next morning, leaving them with the spermatozoa overnight. I turned off the tap then left the laboratory.

Next morning, as usual, I left Gough Way. I did not expect any kind of success to await me in that culture dish. Yet, when I looked, to my delight, one spermatozoon had passed through the outer membrane of an egg. Sperm and egg had not fused – so it was not a complete fertilization. It was enormously encouraging though, for a first attempt. Little did I suspect then that it would be several years before I would see another egg like it.

In the evening I told Ruth what had happened. 'Of course,' I
continued, 'maybe the conditions were too artificial.' Perhaps, in
some way, I had accidentally damaged the outer membrane of
the egg – making it more permeable to the sperm? Perhaps, after
all, only uterine spermatozoa would really do the trick? Either
way I was even more committed to working with the human
egg. More than ever I needed human ovarian tissue. And I wasn't
going to get it in any quantity or with any regularity at
Cambridge.

'Write to Victor McKusick,' suggested Ruth.

Victor lately had taken an interest in my work. He was a
redoubtable geneticist working on inherited human disorders
such as Mongolism, and he was at the Johns Hopkins Hospital in
Baltimore. That American hospital was large, well known, a
considerable stronghold for medical research. Yes, if I could go
there in the summer for six weeks, I might be able to work with
as much human ovarian tissue as I needed.

Victor McKusick responded affirmatively. He suggested that
the most suitable people for me to work with at the Johns
Hopkins Hospital would be the husband and wife team of
gynaecologists, Professor Georgeanna and Howard Jones. The
Ford Foundation also liked my proposal and gave me a grant to
work in Baltimore for six weeks. So that July in 1965, Ruth drove
me to London's Heathrow to see me off.

'Next time there's a chance to go to the USA,' I told Ruth,
'you'll come. I promise.'

I flew off to Baltimore excited at the prospect of six weeks'
research and guilty that I had left Ruth alone in Cambridge
looking after all the family. The very first night Victor had
arranged a dinner party, and of course he had invited my new
collaborators-to-be, Georgeanna and Howard Jones. Victor had
warned them what I was up to. Yet, as I outlined my ideas in
more detail to all three, I once again witnessed the dubious
countenance, the pursed lips. They rallied at last. With relief I
heard Howard Jones say, 'We'll do all we can to help.'

And they did. I was to share pieces of ovarian tissue with the
pathologists and my work started within the week. At last I had
enough human oocytes for careful and considered study. After
two weeks I had no doubts at all about the ripening programme
of the human egg. It took thirty-six hours exactly. All the
difficulties of the preceding years were resolved and I watched

once more those chromosomes marching through the eggs, this time in black and white, half of them moving into the first polar body. I telephoned Ruth regularly to see how she was getting on and to tell her of my progress. Our family were fine it seemed – thriving without me. 'I'm fine too,' I told Ruth. 'I'm going to try fertilization *in vitro* next week.'

I did not succeed, during the next month in Baltimore, in fertilizing one single egg. First I tried adding spermatozoa, as I had in Cambridge, to the human eggs in a culture fluid. This time I drew a blank. So perhaps orthodox opinion was correct after all? Spermatozoa did need, presumably, to be in contact with the secretions of the female reproductive tract. So we collected living spermatozoa from the cervix of some of Howard's patients soon after they had had sexual intercourse with their husbands. These spermatozoa I transferred to the oocytes in the laboratory. Once again, no luck. The eggs remained stubbornly unfertilized. I did not know then that the cervix of the womb was probably the wrong site for spermatozoa to ripen.

We attempted all kinds of manoeuvres. We made our culture fluids resemble the female reproductive tract by adding very small pieces of human uterus or Fallopian tube; we placed some human eggs into the tubes of rabbits then injected into the same lumen a few human spermatozoa also, hoping that the rabbits' Fallopian tubes would be a suitable environment for human fertilization. All these manoeuvres failed. Finally, we tried to fertilize human eggs in the Fallopian tubes of rhesus monkeys – Howard performing the necessary surgery and collecting the eggs twelve to twenty-four hours later. Again without success.

'At least it's a change operating on monkeys rather than on patients,' Howard said drily.

Those weeks in Johns Hopkins were decisive for me. Though we had failed to fertilize one single human egg, I was not deterred. I felt confident I could solve that problem eventually. Why, I had only just begun. I would just have to go down the road that beckoned me. At Cambridge there were other projects, other pathways, but the way ahead for me was clear. Would Alan Parkes and others in Cambridge fully understand my commitment? I thought of those lines by the American poet, Robert Frost:

> Two roads diverged in a wood, and I –
> I took the one less traveled by,
> And that has made all the difference.

As I boarded the Pan Am plane for home, for some reason I felt exultant.

8
Eureka
Robert Edwards

When I returned to Cambridge I found Ruth pale. She had only just overcome a particularly pernicious attack of influenza. It seemed that when I had spoken to her on the phone and asked how she was, and she had replied, as always, 'Fine,' she had a raging fever. The stoical selflessness of women! It was late summer. In the green quadrangles of the Colleges, or on the Backs, there were tourists from America, from Germany, from Japan, from all over the world, and cameras clicked, clicked.

Back home, my first task was to write up all the data on ripening human ova and submit it for publication in the medical press. I was keen to report our Baltimore work and eventually I submitted the human results to the *Lancet*. This was pioneer work and I was bursting with enthusiasm as I parcelled up the manuscript, the illustrations, the photographs. I frankly expected my paper to make a tremendous impact – not least on my colleagues.

A few evenings later we were invited for sherry at Alan Parkes's place. I told him something of my work at Baltimore and what I now, with certainty, wanted to do. As usual, in his deep croaky voice, he was encouraging and sceptical at the same time. Then he turned the conversation to a favourite topic of his – the coming population explosion. 'Pretty anti-social of you having five babies,' he teased Ruth.

The letter from the *Lancet* stunned me. The editor could not see the point of my work. All those complex references to chromosomes, oocytes, and speculations about curing infertility. Was it relevant to the *Lancet*? I have seldom felt so deflated. I took the bull by the horns and phoned him. I asked him as diplomatically as possible why he had misread it.

'It's rather long,' he said.

'I'll shorten it,' I said.

'I'd also like to suggest certain changes,' he said.

'Certainly,' I said.

I wanted my paper published. I accepted all his suggestions, every one, and at last he did publish it. I was delighted and indeed I am still proud of that article in the *Lancet*. Many of its prophecies have now come true and the article was read not only by my colleagues. On 7 November 1965 I picked up the *Sunday Times* from the doormat outside 48 Gough Way. On one side of the front page was the headline: SMITH TURNS DOWN WILSON AND SAYS 'I BLAME YOU.' I had begun to read about the problem in Rhodesia when I noticed the headline on the other side of the front page: BIRTHS MAY BE BY PROXY. Underneath it my own name featured in a story about 'experiments reminiscent of Aldous Huxley's *Brave New World*'.

Though my work on human eggs once more came to a temporary halt, the next few months' research in Cambridge proved to be particularly fruitful. It had occurred to me that, once the problem of human fertilization *in vitro* was solved, the sex of the embryos could be identified at a very early stage by examination of their chromosomes, and that it would be possible therefore to choose whether the mother gave birth to a boy or a girl. At first, animal husbandry would benefit. Farm animals could be induced to superovulate, their fertilized eggs removed, examined to see what sex they were, and only the ova of one or the other sex replaced into the womb of the mother animal.

In man, certain diseases could perhaps be reduced. Certain genetic disorders are sex-linked – they occur almost entirely in males – the blood condition called haemophilia for instance; also one of the muscular dystrophies; and certain enzyme-deficiency diseases too. So by preselecting the sex of the future baby – girls only – such diseases could be eliminated; a benefit not only to the next generation but to the human race for years to come. Of course, there would be debate about the ethics of such a plan – there would be objections – but I dismissed these for the time being and worked with rabbit embryos to see whether theory could become practice. Despite the microscopic size of a rabbit embryo at five days – at this stage the embryo is called a blastocyst – I found I could remove a piece from it. Examining this piece allowed me to identify the future sex of the blastocyst. Most interestingly the blastocyst, as I was to discover later with one of my students, continued to grow normally despite having lost that very tiny section of itself. Indeed, inside the womb of the mother, it developed into a normal baby rabbit.

This was a very fruitful period in my scientific research, working on embryos, on immunology and on human eggs. Alan Henderson and I postulated a theory to explain the origin of Down's syndrome (Mongolism), based on an analysis of those ripening mouse eggs, and it still stands today. If we are right, there is virtually no hope of averting the formation of these and other embryos with unbalanced chromosomes, sad to say.

I was travelling extensively too, mostly to discuss immunology and reproduction, and it was at one of these meetings in Venice, organized by the Ford Foundation, that I met Gregory Pincus for the last time and we came to our inevitable battle about ripening human eggs. I had met Pincus two or three times previously. He was one of the hardest men of science I ever met. He had a direct manner, asked blunt questions of each lecturer, and displayed obvious disbelief if he didn't share the same opinion. We got on well until I found his work impossible to repeat. I couldn't accept his results and he didn't believe mine, and we were inevitably drawn into open conflict. It was rough going, at least for me, but I was determined not to be browbeaten. There had been some Anglo-American rivalry the previous day, when I had been unable to accept some American work on the mode of action of the intrauterine contraceptive device. Some needle persisted, and when it was my turn to lecture on ripening eggs, Pincus was among those who had a shot at me. Perhaps I convinced him in the end, for we got on well, if all too briefly, from then until his untimely death.

My work on animals was only a stop-gap until I could work again with human eggs. Another opportunity arose in the summer of 1966 to work with gynaecologists in the USA – this time in Chapel Hill, North Carolina. As promised, I took Ruth and the five girls with me. My plan was to continue where I had left off a year earlier in Baltimore. I needed to collect human spermatozoa from a woman's reproductive tract before using them in attempts to fertilize the eggs. I decided to construct a very small chamber which I could fill with spermatozoa before inserting it into the womb. This chamber was lined with a porous membrane that would allow uterine secretions to pass into it but would not let sperms escape.

'Are you sure they won't escape?' asked Ruth.

'Sure,' I said.

Once again my American colleagues gave me their full collaboration. What a business it all was: collecting pieces of human ovarian tissue, ripening the eggs, collecting spermatozoa and putting them into the little chambers, and then finding a volunteer who would allow this chamber to be inserted into her womb. I have cause to be grateful to those ladies of Chapel Hill who volunteered in sufficient numbers for me to continue my research. The chamber with its busy spermatozoa would be inserted at night and removed the next morning and I must confess that I had many a sleepless night fearing the chamber would burst inside the uterus, releasing the spermatozoa with disastrous results.

'You said you were sure they couldn't escape,' Ruth said.

'I am sure,' I replied.

'Then go to sleep, for heaven's sake,' Ruth insisted.

Fortunately the membrane held. The living spermatozoa were added next day to ripe eggs in the culture dish. But again and again there was no fertilization. It was a pleasant summer interlude for me and my family, but when we returned to Cambridge it seemed I had come to an impasse. I could not think of any practical way, other than those home-made, semi-permeable chambers, of letting spermatozoa be in contact with the secretions of the female tract. I could hardly expect any woman to submit to an operation so that some time after intercourse spermatozoa could be collected from her Fallopian tubes. If only there was some simple way of doing that!

There was. I discovered this to be so one autumn day in 1967 and, like Archimedes, I wanted to shout out, 'Eureka!' I always kept a careful eye on the medical and scientific journals. Whenever I was free I would go to one or another library, for Cambridge is an ideal place for browsing. That afternoon, I glanced at a journal and read about something called laparoscopy. It was a method whereby the inside of the abdomen could be explored without resorting to a major operation. The instrument, the laparoscope, could be inserted at the umbilicus by a surgeon trained in the technique with the minimum of disturbance to the patient. Indeed the patient need only be in hospital for thirty-six hours. It all seemed too good to be true. I was looking for just this expertise. The article was by a gynaecologist called Patrick Steptoe who, it seemed, could through laparoscopy collect solutions – or indeed, spermatozoa – from the Fallopian tubes quite simply. Steptoe, what a curious name. The only Steptoe I had heard of was in the television comedy series then popular in Britain called *Steptoe and Son*. This real Steptoe was working at Oldham General Hospital. Why wasn't this gynaecologist attached to one of the fine teaching hospitals rather than practising in the backwater of a once-prosperous Lancashire mill town?

I could not resist telephoning him. 'Steptoe here,' a deep voice responded. I told him my name, my credentials such as they were, my curiosity about laparoscopy and how deeply interesting I had found his article. I asked him further questions about its possibilities. He replied enthusiastically and eventually, encouraged, I explained what I wanted and why. 'Ripen eggs in culture fluids, collect spermatozoa from the Fallopian tubes . . . .' My usual speech, but would I get the usual response?

I was talking in Cambridge. He was listening to me in Oldham. Did his countenance change, did that old apprehensive look appear in his eyes? I don't know. When he spoke there was no audible tremor in his voice. 'Let's have a try,' he said. 'Let's see what we can do.' I promised to call him back.

Oldham – that was a hell of a way from Cambridge. I looked at the map. Though only 165 miles as the crow flies, it was considerably further by the twisting roads. And when I reached Oldham what facilities would be there? General hospitals were not equipped as research laboratories. Oldham General would be no exception. I talked the whole thing over with Ruth. I knew that any collaboration I had with a gynaecologist at Oldham while I lived in Cambridge would present a formidable logistic problem and would disrupt my family life. No wonder I hesitated.

'I'll be absent from the family and from the research here in Cambridge for long periods of time maybe,' I told Ruth.

Ruth felt that I should try all the same – though she knew

that I would have to drive fast to Oldham when ovarian tissue
became available, usually at very short notice. Also, I would
have to wait in the hospital for thirty six hours for the human
eggs to ripen, persuading volunteer patients waiting for laparoscopy to have intercourse so that Steptoe could then collect
the sperms from the Fallopian tubes.

'It's too much,' I said. 'I would have to wait even longer –
yet another twelve hours or more – to see if fertilization
occurred *in vitro*.'

'If only human eggs were like those of mice and ripened in
twelve hours on the dot, that would simplify it a bit!' sighed
Ruth.

I sat tight and continued my work on the sex identification
of rabbit embryos, collaborating with one of my first Ph.D
students, Richard Gardner. My thoughts often strayed to
Oldham, but each time I thought about it I decided the
problems were too enormous. But then I happened to attend
a conference on gynaecology. It was at the Royal Society of
Medicine in London's Wimpole Street. Sitting in the rows of
green chairs, facing the raised platform and the lectern, were
many distinguished gynaecologists and endocrinologists. Next
to the chairman was the speaker, leaning towards the micro-
phone, and behind and above him was a small cinema-like
screen. One of the topics discussed was the disadvantage of
the fertility drugs for they led too often to multipregnancies
(as had happened to my mice in Edinburgh). 'If only the
ovaries could be inspected easily beforehand,' the speaker
continued, 'then we would have advance warning of multipregnancies. We'd see how many eggs were growing. Perhaps
the new method of laparoscopy could be of use here?'

People lolled in their chairs. It was an august gathering and
the chairman had no need to disturb anybody by bringing his
wooden mallet down sharply and shouting, 'Order, Order.'
But suddenly a distinguished-looking gentleman, sitting in
front of me, rose to his feet.

'No,' he said, dogmatically. 'Laparoscopy is of no use whatsoever. It is impossible to visualize the ovary using that
technique. I've tried it.'

He was suggesting it was just a gynaecological gimmick,
and I began to think that perhaps it was as well that I had not
committed myself to Oldham when, at the back of the hall, a

thick-set, grey-haired man leapt to his feet, evidently impatient with the speaker. He did not actually say, 'Rubbish' but his remarks were pungent and direct. Forcefully, he recounted how, through laparoscopy, not only the ovaries could be seen, but also the Fallopian tubes and other parts of the reproductive tract. 'Indeed,' he continued, 'the whole abdominal cavity can be inspected. You are hopelessly wrong. I carry out laparoscopy routinely every day – many times over. It is simple and it only takes me a matter of minutes.'

This obviously was *the* Patrick Steptoe of Oldham General Hospital. I felt immediately that here was a man I could trust and respect and work with. He knew his mind. He was utterly convincing and he offered to demonstrate, on the screen, the slides he had brought along to substantiate his claims. Afterwards, in the foyer, near the marble columns of the Royal Society of medicine, I approached him.

'You're Patrick Steptoe,' I said.

'Yes.'

'I'm Bob Edwards. Six months ago we spoke on the telephone.'

'You've never called me back,' he accused me.

Even as he began to speak I wondered what kind of a man Steptoe was – what was his background, and why had he ended up in Oldham of all places?

9

To Oldham then I Came

Patrick Steptoe

While Bob Edwards was a student at Bangor University, uncertain of his future and facing the wrong direction, I was already 38 years of age, a practising gynaecologist, living with my wife Sheena, my four-year-old daughter Sally, and our baby son Andrew, in a London flat near Highgate Village. If I had known Bob then, he would have thought me affluent and settled, a man who knew where he was going.

I was going to Oldham. The job at Highgate was coming to an end. Some months earlier, in 1951, I had obtained the Edinburgh Fellowship of the Royal College of Surgeons, so I was now ready to take up a consultant post. It was far from easy to become established in London. Four hundred of my contemporaries were also competing to become consultants in the metropolitan area.

'London's not the only place in Britain,' Sheena had said.

So, eventually, I applied for the Oldham job. Kathleen Harding, my immediate chief – an excellent clinician at a time when there were few women consultants in gynaecology – had kindly said that she would miss us, Sheena and me, and had invited us once more to dinner in her maisonette right at the top of a house in Harley Street.

She was in her early sixties and had had for some time a special interest in family planning and infertility. I had learned so much from her. Before she trained me I'm afraid I had not treated infertile couples very well. As was customary in those post-war years I took a history, discussed coital habits, chatted a little about fertility and ovulation, and then admitted the lady into hospital for a D and C – a diagnostic curettage of the uterus.

Once in hospital the patient would also be tested to see whether her Fallopian tubes were obstructed. I would do this by using a gas insufflation machine or by injecting the tubes and uterus with an opaque dye and then X raying them. If nothing was found to be wrong the lady would be reassured, patted on the back, and told to come back in two years' time should she not become pregnant meanwhile. Her husband was rarely investigated at all. Often, after two more years of infertility, the patient would return and be readmitted to hospital for a further bout of inadequate investigation. Kathleen Harding changed these procedures for me.

As we drove to her maisonette I thought how, thanks to Kathleen, the experience I had gained during the last two years would be invaluable in Oldham. Through her I had become much more aware than I had been as a student at St George's Hospital that infertility was a complaint of two people, not of one – a complaint which could cause life-long unhappiness. To some it became an obsession. Sometimes it disrupted what otherwise might have been an amiable marriage. There were men who, fearful that they were sterile, became impotent. There were women who, desperate, tried folk remedies, prayed for long hours in a darkened room, or visited special shrines. Kathleen Harding did not know all the answers – in 1951 less was known generally about the mechanisms of ovulation, tubal function, spermatozoal and hormone activity – but she kindled in me a strong wish to learn more about the mystery of infertility problems.

If someone asked me, 'Why did you become a gynaecologist?' I suppose I would have to reply, 'I don't know.' Perhaps there were many reasons. I liked women. All gynaecologists do – otherwise they would hardly be very good gynaecologists. My very name, Patrick, was chosen after the doctor who delivered me that night in 1913, in Witney, a small Oxfordshire market town, near the Cotswold Hills. And my mother who had eight children, who was very conscious of the rights of women and the wrongs done to them, and who found time to organize the local Mothers' Union, the Infant Welfare Clinics, and clubs for elderly people, had always gently suggested that one day I might be able to help them.

These were some of the reasons. There were others. When I had been a medical student before the war, before I qualified and joined the Navy, antibiotics had not been discovered and the wards of St George's Hospital were crammed with people suffering acute infections such as pneumonia, meningitis, septicaemia. There were too many patients that one could do nothing worthwhile for. There were too many people in pain and dying. In the neurological ward so much was academic: long hours of investigation and examination to prove, say, that a patient suffered from syringomyelia or some other disease of the nervous system, and then not to be able to offer any treatment for it. How refreshing, in contrast, to deliver a healthy baby to a delighted woman! That was one reason why I thought about becoming a gynaecologist.

Then there were certain dramatic cases I shall remember all my life. For instance, a lovely red-haired girl was admitted into the wards because she had been the victim of a septic criminal abortion done in Finsbury Park. She developed tetanus, from which she died. First she displayed lock-jaw. The disease progressed so that she suffered stiffness and rigidity of the neck, back, abdomen and the extremities. The involvement of her facial muscles caused her to grin grotesquely. Terrible spasms would begin as the result of the slightest stimuli – a jarring of her bed, a draught of cold air, a noise of any kind, a light switched on in the corridor when the door opened. At her post mortem I felt angry before her body on the slab – her beautiful figure, the pale face at last at rest, the striking red hair – angry as I observed the pathologist demonstrate how her abortion had been cruelly botched.

Soon I was parking the car in Harley Street. And so, that August evening in 1951, Sheena and I went up to Kathleen's maisonette to take our leave.

Kathleen was then a grey-haired, bespectacled, slightly plump spinster who wore rather mannish suits. I was always surprised how pleasantly feminine her rooms were. That evening after dinner I sat at her piano, as usual, and played while she sang Schubert songs in her modulated voice.

'Did Patrick tell you of his career as a cinema accompanist when he was thirteen?' Sheena asked.

When a boy in Witney, I had helped the resident pianist at the local Palace cinema by playing, during matinées, the incidental music for the silent films of Tom Mix, Harold Lloyd, Ramon Novarro, Rudolph Valentino. A few years later I played the organ at the local St Mary's Church. The weight on the fingers when the manuals were coupled together with full organ was very heavy, and because I spent hours and hours each week at this organ my hands and fingers became very strong. They still are. Perhaps those early years of learning dexterity and needing strength and sensitivity helped my surgical technique. I like to think that this is the case.

'Sheena will miss London,' Kathleen said just before we left. Sheena had trained as an actress and was employed by the BBC. But we would return from time to time. Oldham was not the end of the world. Of course, during the war I had been a prisoner of war in Italy for two years. After that, Sheena suggested, Oldham, whatever it was like, would be heaven.

'All he likes most,' she said, 'the smell of hospitals, the gleaming corridors, the atmosphere, the team work, he'll find in Lancashire as well as anywhere else. And there's music, as the saying goes, wherever he goes!'

A month later we travelled to Oldham. I was to start work on 1 October 1951 on maximum part-time sessions for an annual salary of £1800. We were taken aback by the unpleasing appearance of the industrial north. But we found a pleasant, large comfortable house in Rochdale, six miles away from the main hospital where I was to work. And there was so much work to do. They needed a gynaecologist desperately. I had never seen women with such enormous tumours, such degrees of uterine prolapse. So many patients! It would take me years to work through the back-log. Here was a chance indeed to uphold the rights of women and alleviate, as my mother would have wished, some of the wrongs done to them.

At first, there were many obstacles put in my way but one of my mother's mottoes had been, 'Obstacles which you meet are really opportunities in disguise.' For the next few years I was to find myself heavily involved in major surgery and obstetrics. Kathleen Harding would have been appalled by the inadequacies of our management of infertility and, indeed, also of fertility. I did not have enough time. There were priorities to consider. A woman saying, 'Doctor, we've been trying to have a baby for years without success,' had, it seemed, less claim on my attention than those who needed urgent operations. But I brooded about it and did what I could and even managed to establish Family Planning Clinics. I was over-worked, aware of the deficiencies in our service to patients, but I was beginning to organize things, to enlist more help gradually. I even began to have some weekends free!

10
If Only
Patrick Steptoe

Though, very occasionally, I brooded on my failure to have
gained a consultant post in London – at my own hospital, St
George's – we were content with life in the industrial north-west
of England. We would not have willingly exchanged our settled
provincial way of life for one more apparently glittering in
London. Lancashire has much to offer: accessible and charming
countryside, regular concerts in Manchester, cricket to watch at
Old Trafford, first-class theatre in Oldham itself, and at weekends
I was able to go sailing. The years passed quickly and in what
seemed no time at all, our youngsters had begun to grow up.
Above all, I was finding my work more and more satisfying.

I now had very capable help from Frank da Cunha, a gynaecologist of Portuguese origin, educated in England, and some five
years my junior. There was but one snag. Frank was a very strict
Catholic and so had theological reasons for not being interested
in investigating certain problems of fertility. Nearly all the
fertility and infertility cases, all the necessary abortions and
sterilizations, were saved for me. I did not complain: I was
interested in such cases but since our gynaecological and obstetric
National Health unit served a population of 300,000 people I
continued to remain extremely busy.

One problem that exercised me regularly was the laparotomies
I had to undertake. A laparotomy is an operation in which the
abdominal cavity of the patient is opened up primarily for
diagnostic reasons – so that the surgeon can directly visualize and
feel the tissues and organs laid bare. As a result he may discover
that all is organically normal or he may be able to pinpoint
accurately the source of all the patient's troubles and symptoms.
Such laparotomy operations, although surgically simple, are not
lightly undertaken. But if the case history, the signs and symp-

toms themselves, the special tests, X rays and so on, cannot together point to a conclusive diagnosis, then the doctor may be left with no alternative.

It was not that laparotomies did harm. Simply, the patients were grossly inconvenienced by them. Besides, these exploratory operations showed too often that our pre-operative provisional diagnoses were wrong. In investigating sterility, in particular, I have found that certain other diagnostic aids – curettage, X rays, tubal insufflation, hormone estimations – could actually be misleading. So I had to rely on laparotomy too frequently.

I often wished that there was a safe and efficient means to peer into the abdomen without having to resort to a laparotomy incision. Often I thought, 'If only . . . .' For instance, early in 1957, I decided that one of our own nursing sisters needed a laparotomy. She had originally consulted me because of an infertility problem.

'How old are you?'

'Twenty-eight.'

'How long have you been married?'

'Six years.'

She had been trying for a baby without success. Soon after that first consultation it so happened that my patient missed a period. When she was four weeks overdue she began to experience a tight, unilateral pain in her abdomen. She consulted me again. 'The pain waxes and wanes,' she told me. I admitted her to our unit of course. She had a vague swelling.

There was no sign of an infection: her white blood cell count – raised when there is an inflammation – was normal. Nor did she have any real anaemia. *Was this an ectopic pregnancy?* I wondered. In other words, had she become pregnant and the fertilized ovum become lodged in one of her Fallopian tubes to grow there rather than in the uterus? Other investigations were inconclusive. Even the pregnancy test – in those days not so accurate as now – was equivocal.

I stood by her bedside and said, 'We'll wait a little while. We'll watch how things go.' She was a sallow-faced young woman who wore her dark hair in a bun. She trusted me implicitly. Her intelligent eyes met mine.

'Will I need a laparotomy, Mr Steptoe?' she asked.

I hesitated. 'It may come to that,' I confessed.

Her pain became worse. We could wait no longer. Again I

wished I could peer into her abdomen without doing a laparotomy. Again I looked at the X ray plates. Again I decided they
were of no help. I had no choice finally. In the event, I discovered
she had a *corpus luteum* cyst. The cyst would have withered
away on its own and no surgical intervention would have been
necessary if I had known the diagnosis beforehand. I shook my
head.

After I returned from the operating theatre I recalled, not for
the first time, a paper I had read, after the war, by a surgeon
working in Bristol which had been published in 1925. His name
was Rendle Short. I had slotted this paper in my mind. He had
distended the abdomen with air, under local anaesthesia, and had
inserted into the abdomen a cystoscope – an instrument normally
used for visualizing the interior of the bladder. Through peering
into this cystoscope he had been able to recognize cancer nodules
in the liver, tuberculosis, peritonitis, tumours in the pelvis and
ectopic pregnancies. There were dangers in such a crude envi-
sioning of the abdominal cavity. But in the 1940s Albert Decker,
a New York gynaecologist, had perfected the instrument and
used his 'telescope' to peer into the female pelvis. He approached
the abdominal cavity through the vagina – inserting the instrument between the back of the uterus and the front of the rectum.
He performed all this using only a local anaesthetic. This procedure was called 'culdoscopy'. The trouble was that women were
required to take up a most undignified position – the knee-chest
posture – and also there were accidents when gynaecologists
other than Decker attempted it. Culdoscopy certainly had not
found favour in Britain. But as I said to Sheena, 'Our infertile
patients are not getting a fair crack of the whip. I feel I must do
something about this.'

I was thinking that, despite its disfavour in Britain, I should
learn more about culdoscopy. In the summer of 1958 I had an
opportunity to do exactly that at an International Congress in
Montreal. Anxious to learn more, ready to be persuaded of the
value of culdoscopy, I flew to Canada. There I met Professor
Jeffcoate of Liverpool – the only British gynaecologist who was
enthusiastic about culdoscopy. But after the congress I saw the
culdoscope in use in hospitals in Boston and in New York. I was
not impressed. There were dangers of introducing infection into
the abdominal cavity from the vagina – and possible injuries also
to the rectum.

I had heard and read of alternative methods of viewing the abdominal cavity developed by Raoul Palmer in Paris. His approach was to insert the viewing instrument – the laparoscope – into the abdominal cavity at the navel. The instrument worked like a telescope, with an eye-piece to look through and with a lens inside the abdomen which permitted a view of the body organs. On returning home, I said to Sheena, 'I want to go to Paris to see Raoul Palmer.'

Sheena looked puzzled. 'Who's he?' she asked. I explained that he was Director of Infertility at a Paris hospital and why I wanted to witness his pioneer work.

'Off you go then,' Sheena said.

I discovered how laparoscopy gave a magnificent view inside the female pelvis provided it was first filled with a balloon of harmless gas – carbon dioxide. The difficulty was that the electric lamp became hot quickly or would break so the whole procedure had to be performed very rapidly. It was a smash-and-grab surgical procedure. Yet I was very impressed by Raoul Palmer and his tall Dutch wife, Elizabeth, who assisted him.

When I learnt that Palmer was to read a paper at an Amsterdam Congress in 1959, I was on my travels again. There I saw a film on laparoscopy by Hans Frangenheim who was an assistant in Wuppertal, West Germany, to Professor Anselmino. Frangenheim had the advantage of being backed by the lens-manufacturing companies of Germany so his laparoscope was more refined than the one used in Paris. I decided it was time to introduce laparoscopy into my unit. Our department, by now, had gained an excellent reputation in the Manchester area and I received, when I spoke of my intentions, immediate and unreserved support from my Hospital Management Committee.

So, shortly, with the new German equipment they allowed me to buy, I was practising my technique on fresh cadavers awaiting post mortem in the mortuary. At lunch-time, off I would go to the mortuary with a newly qualified young houseman to assist me. Beforehand, of course, I had to ask permission to practise laparoscopy on the dead by approaching the distressed and distracted relatives. What a business that was! And how macabre visiting the mortuary when others were away, all eating their lunch! After a period of four or five months, having practised on some thirty corpses, I felt I was ready to try out a laparoscopy examination on a live patient.

One of our physicians at Oldham was a rather tall Yorkshire-man, John Hirst. He was a man who never minced his words. Now he referred a nurse to me who had unexplained abdominal pain. Again the investigations were inconclusive. So here was another nurse who seemed a candidate for exploratory surgery.

'I would like to try laparoscopy on this patient,' I told John Hirst.

'Laparotomy?'

'No, laparoscopy.'

We explained it to the nurse who seemed glad to undergo a laparoscopy – she knew it would be much less gruelling than a laparotomy. Maybe I was nervous working on a live patient rather than on one of those female corpses. In any event, the procedure did not work. I failed. The lights were lowered in the operating theatre but though facilitated by the semi-darkness I did not see the organs as I had hoped and as I had done in the dead bodies. This was a smash-and-grab where nobody went away with anything. I felt terribly discouraged.

'You must try again,' said John Hirst.

'I don't think so,' I said. 'Besides, the patient wouldn't want to go through that again.'

'I'll talk to her,' said John Hirst masterfully.

When in certain moods I would frequently find myself at the piano. That evening, at home, was no exception. For two years I had hoped to introduce into our unit a method to improve our diagnostic methods, especially in cases of infertility. I had studied culdoscopy and laparoscopy. I had gone to congresses all over the world, to hospitals in America and Europe. I had practised diligently on those dead ladies in the mortuary. And now I had come to this blind end. I put down the piano lid and thought of our old family saying that I had heard my mother repeat so often: 'Obstacles which you meet are really opportunities in disguise.'

John Hirst persuaded the nurse to allow me to repeat the laparoscopy. 'So it's up to you now, Patrick,' he said.

That second attempt was most successful. I was able to see clearly the size, texture and colour of the whole uterus. It was normal. I inspected each broad ligament, ovary and Fallopian tube. They were normal. Wherever I looked I saw plainly normal tissue, normal organs. There was no surgical cause here for my patient's pain. Now she would need no exploratory operation – no operation at all.

That nurse was grateful to me, but I was even more grateful to her. Since that first failure I have been engaged in a long career of laparoscopy and I have never failed since.

Moreover I was soon able to start using a new equipment invented by French scientists and developed by Palmer. He had a thin rod of quartz incorporated in the laparoscope which was able to carry light cooled by an electric fan from outside the body to the tip of the instrument within the abdomen. So intense was light thus distributed that Palmer was able to take colour photographs of the condition found in the pelvis for permanent records. No lamps inside the tummy any more.

Confronted with patients who are, gynaecologically speaking, an apparent puzzle, I have not had to say, as I used to, at first, in Oldham, 'If only . . . .'

11

Laparoscopy Comes of Age

Patrick Steptoe

Since my first laparoscopy on John Hirst's patient, I had repeated the procedure in a further 126 cases. I felt strongly now that abdominal exploration as a means of establishing a true diagnosis was an excessive surgical act, involving sacrifices on the part of the patient which were scarcely justified.

By now, I had become accustomed to the delicate instruments which are used to move and examine the internal organs. They were no wider than a narrow knitting needle and could be pushed easily through the abdominal wall. They had a delicate, finger-tip control which enabled me to make adjustments to the organs, or to excise samples of tissue literally at the flick of one of my fingers.

Using these methods I had developed ways of exploring the Fallopian tubes, of obtaining specimens from inside the abdominal cavity, and of introducing into them prepared cultures containing spermatozoa. It was all so simple that the patient needed only three small clips when the laparoscopy was over and these were removed next day just before she went home.

This procedure was indicated when the couple had no babies because of the husband's very low sperm count. I reasoned that in these cases, if I introduced the spermatozoa into the lumen of his wife's Fallopian tubes conception was more likely to occur. It was a question of giving those rare sperms a better chance to reach their goal. Alas, my attempts at fertilization by this method were not successful.

In November 1964 the first International Symposium on Gynaecological Laparoscopy was held in Palermo, the capital of Sicily, and I was invited to submit a paper through the agency of Raoul Palmer. That Congress proved to be a most significant event in the practice of gynaecology throughout the world.

In the course of my own paper I felt I had to apologize for the
slowness with which the value of laparoscopy was being accepted
in the United Kingdom and I pledged myself to try to convert as
many of my colleagues as possible to recognize the method as an
essential technique. I spoke of the progress in my own unit
where, in the three-and-a-half years that had elapsed since I first
started to use the laparoscope, 4615 patients had been admitted to
the beds for which I was responsible, and of these I had considered
laparoscopy necessary and helpful in 126 cases, an incidence of
2.7 per cent.

I had come to the symposium determined to learn more, and
I did. We were told of an amazing technical advance in the
lighting of the laparoscope from the Storz Instrument Company
and the Richard Wolf Instrument Company of West Germany
working with Hans Frangenheim.

Together they had developed a laparoscope in which the light
was conducted from a mirror projection lamp of low voltage
along a flexible-fibre glass guide. Professor Harold Hopkins of
Reading University's Department of Physics had invented the
fibre-optic system twelve years earlier. He and his associate,
Kapany, had put together, in a bundle, some hundreds of very
fine glass fibres with marvellous precision. As a result the bundle,
of a length say of one metre, was capable of transmitting light
from one end of its length to the other. Moreover, if an intense
source of light was bounced in at one end of the fibre-optic
bundle by means of a mirror, the heat produced could be
dissipated by a motorized fan by the time the light had reached
the other end of the cable. Alas, English instrument makers had
not recognized the fibre-optic system as an important innovation.
It was left to the Germans to develop it. By a clever system of
prisms and mirrors an intense beam of light was produced at the
end of a telescope which, hey presto!, had no electrical connec-
tions and was cool. No longer, with such an invention, would
laparoscopy be a swift, smash-and-grab affair. Now it could be
employed in a leisurely manner so that accurate diagnoses could
be made, particularly in the female pelvis. (This same fibre-optic
system is now used for viewing all kinds of cavities, not only
those within the human body, but in engines and machines also.)

At Palermo, I had a conversation with Dr Raoul Palmer of
particular importance to me. Palmer – Frangenheim too – had
been interested in developing laparoscopy not only as a diagnostic

tool but also to carry out certain operative procedures. One of these involved the possibility of sterilizing women whose fertility was already fulfilled by the destruction of a small piece of each Fallopian tube by means of an electric current.

'I can't do it often enough in France,' Raoul said, 'as it's a Catholic country. And Hans Frangenheim has difficulties, too, because he's working in a Catholic region of Germany. But you, Patrick, live in England, and you could work unimpeded.'

He was correct. In England, sterilization by open operation was already being offered to women on both medical and social grounds. I was in the fortunate position of being able to develop laparoscopic methods of sterilization freely. How much simpler and less troublesome for the patient than having to undergo the present operation! It meant now that women could be taken into hospital for a few hours and sterilized by laparoscopic methods in a few minutes. They would be fully recovered in less than two days.

Back in Oldham I used the laparoscope for sterilization as well as for diagnostic purposes. I performed the first ever fifty cases sterilized in this fashion and I continued to develop the laparoscopic methods freely. Since then some 40 million women in the world have had sterilization by this method. This has often been paraphrased: 'Palmer introduced us to laparoscopy, Frangenheim developed the instrumentation but Steptoe taught us how to use it.' I certainly wrote scientific papers and published them in the journals in order to report what I had done and to persuade other gynaecologists in Britain of the value of laparoscopy for their patients. Sadly, the majority of gynaecologists, impressed with the sterilization reports, interpreted this as the main indication for laparoscopy, failing to recognize for some years its imperative place in diagnosis, especially in the field of infertility.

During 1965 and 1966 I sat down to write a textbook on laparoscopy in gynaecology. I hoped that this book, which was published in 1967, would convince my British colleagues particularly of the many valuable indications for the use of laparoscopy.

Just before my textbook was published, one evening I had a surprising telephone call from a Dr Robert Edwards of Cambridge. He was a scientist studying human ova and embryology and now he was asking me about laparoscopic methods of taking samples from the human Fallopian tubes and ovaries. Apparently he had read one of my published papers on laparoscopy.

'I find your article deeply interesting,' he said.

He spoke swiftly, with a curious northern accent, and was suggesting how fertilization might be effected *in vitro*. It seemed he was asking for my help. 'I'm perfectly willing to help as much as possible,' I finally responded. 'Let's see what we can manage.'

'Thank you,' Robert Edwards said. 'I'll be telephoning you again.'

I put down the phone and stared out of the window. He had not indicated how he was going to put the spermatozoa and eggs together. I wondered about that and thought that I would not mind meeting Dr Edwards to discuss his ideas further. He did not, however, telephone me again as he had promised. Evidently he had had second thoughts.

Early in 1968 I attended a meeting of the Endocrinological and Gynaecological Sections of the Royal Society of Medicine. This meeting took place at the Society in Wimpole Street, London, and because they were to discuss polycystic ovarian disease – a curious disorder of the ovaries associated with lack of menstruation, overweight, hairiness and infertility – I brought down some electrifying colour slides of these disordered ovaries which I had taken through the laparoscope. Most endocrinologists and many gynaecologists were unaware that not only could the laparoscope provide clear naked-eye views of the internal organs but that these could also be photographed and filmed in full colour, such was the brilliance of the Hopkins light system. Indeed, I was able to take better shots inside the abdomen than I could outside with an ordinary camera.

I was sitting next to Professor W. I. C. Morris of the University of Manchester, who had kindly written the foreword to my textbook. We heard some absurd anti-laparoscopy remarks being made. I listened, glowering, to a gynaecologist who had been working in association with the endocrinologist David Ferris, an old friend of mine – years earlier, as students, we had played hockey together. But now his gynaecologist colleague was suggesting that without laparotomy the only way to visualize the ovaries was by X ray examination and I could no longer contain myself. I rose to my feet involuntarily and shouted, '*Non*sense!' There was a sudden silence. I repeated myself. 'Absolute nonsense,' I said. 'You're quite wrong. I carry out laparoscopy regularly each day, many times a day.'

People were murmuring and Professor Morris at my elbow, in

support, called, 'Hear, hear.'

David Ferris intervened coolly. 'Ah yes,' he remarked. 'I thought this might turn out to be a provocative meeting.' There were some 200 or so doctors present. A few of them laughed.

'May I,' I now continued less heatedly, 'prove my point with some colour slides I've brought along with me?'

There was another hush during the showing of these slides and afterwards warm applause. Someone – I believe it was Elliot Philipp, a senior gynaecological colleague from the Royal Northern Hospital, London – stood up and said, 'We must congratulate Mr Steptoe on those beautiful photographs.' I must confess I was feeling pleased with myself, I had come down from Oldham and I had triumphed over these London doctors. Perhaps, deep down, by not getting a consultant post in a London teaching hospital as had been my original ambition, I had felt somewhat rejected and had responded with an unspoken, 'I'll show 'em!' Well, now I had! I did not know that very soon I was to encounter Robert Edwards in the foyer and so for that reason alone I would never forget this particular meeting at the Royal Society of Medicine.

The man who approached me was tall, with dark unruly hair, a head held high and tilted a little backwards, a prominent nose and brown, piercing, intelligent eyes.

'You're Patrick Steptoe,' he pronounced.

'Yes.'

'I'm Bob Edwards. We spoke on the phone six months ago.'

'That's right,' I said. 'But you never called me back.'

After a few minutes' conversation I felt that his scientific approach to infertility problems was harder, more penetrating, than those of practising gynaecologists. As I listened to his proposals about recovering eggs from patients, of possibly placing them with spermatozoa direct into Fallopian tubes, of giving certain hormones and so on, I decided that this was a unique opportunity for me to collaborate closely with a scientist of international repute. He was a scientist, I was a doctor. We both wanted to help people who had seemingly insoluble infertility problems. So why not?

'All the clinical material is centred in Oldham,' I said. 'Cambridge is a long way away.'

'I know,' Robert Edwards said. 'We'd have to set up a small research laboratory in Oldham. Would that be possible?'

'Not impossible,' I responded.

12

The Magic Culture Fluid

Robert Edwards

Patrick Steptoe had been given a small room in the Pathology Department at Oldham which I could turn into a small research laboratory. It was a tiny room, an old store-room, but it would serve my purposes. 'Perhaps Clare will go to Oldham with you and help set it up,' Ruth said. Clare Jackson, an attractive, red-headed young woman, would soon be leaving my laboratory in Cambridge where she was my assistant – but before she quit I was sure she would help me in every way. So when I told her my problem, and how it would take several journeys to fit that small room satisfactorily, I was not surprised when she said, 'When do we go?'

On April Fool Day 1968, she and I carried the equipment to the car: the microscopes and culture fluids and all the apparatus I would need. It was my first trip to Oldham. I did not know then that there would be so much driving ahead of me. From Cambridge to Oldham, from Oldham to Cambridge in the years to come – more than a quarter of a million miles to cover before our goal was reached. That journey proved to be one from Science into Medicine, from the free and easy ways of a Cambridge research lab into a world of patients and nurses and doctors with all their busy concerns, their age-old anxieties and legitimate hopes.

One rainy day I set off alone from Cambridge – the white blossom on the trees wet and bedraggled and the daffodils seemingly dying on their stalks. Patrick had invited me to his house in Rochdale and we would discuss, now that the little research laboratory was fitted, our immediate strategy over a leisurely dinner. Lancashire generally experiences more rain than Cambridge but that afternoon the further north-west I travelled the less cloudy the skies. As I approached Oldham, the sun was totally triumphant, the April sky different hues of blue. Oldham is not the most beautiful of towns but the pleasant spring-time weather made it a place full of welcome.

And Mrs Steptoe welcomed me too. Sheena Steptoe was tall, dark, and dressed in a sophisticated, tasteful way. She took my arm warmly as she led me into her elegant home. The Steptoes occupied one half of a large mansion. There was a feeling of spaciousness and grace about the house – generous windows, settees, soft carpets, a big portrait on the wall of the Steptoe children. And in the sitting room among cool shadows, the grand piano and the harpsichord and bowls of flowers – carnations, daffodils. All around and about the house, through those same generous windows, I was aware of green, expansive lawns It was evident that Patrick Steptoe was used to a more luxurious way of life than I. It made no difference. Patrick knew the world of doctors and I knew the world of scientists. Right from the beginning we recognized exactly our respective tasks, the division of labour. We both could make quick decisions. We both could grasp each other's problems.

'It's a question of taking one step at a time,' I told Patrick. I promised that when he phoned me with the information that, because of essential surgical reasons, he would have some ovarian tissue available, I would immediately drive up from Cambridge. I would be able to start the spare eggs ripening in a culture fluid. So much for the ova, but what about the spermatozoa?

Patrick nodded. 'I'll explain to some of my patients who have been admitted for a hysterectomy what we want to do. Perhaps some of them will volunteer to help us. I feel sure they will.'

It would mean Patrick asking such volunteers to have inter-course with their husbands, then through laparoscopy collecting a few spermatozoa from their Fallopian tubes. All this prior to the hysterectomy, the removal of the uterus, the real reason why these women had been admitted to hospital in the first place.

'Perhaps you could also try placing the ripening eggs and the spermatozoa into the tubes of these patients and then recover them after their hysterectomy,' I suggested.

We discussed other details of how we would proceed. Ethical concerns hardly entered into our conversation. We both knew that about 1.2 per cent or more of women – 4000 to 8000 brides each year in Britain alone – could not conceive because of blocked Fallopian tubes and that more than half of these could not be helped by orthodox therapy. We were also aware that our work would enable us to examine a microscopic human being – one in its very earliest stages of development – and as a result of our scrutiny we could well gain new knowledge about genetic disorders. Our hopes were high, our resolve firm, our agreement with each other total.

My journeys to Oldham became more purposeful in that I had to arrive at a certain time. Often I would leave Cambridge at 6 a.m. because of an operation being scheduled in Oldham mid-morning. Now in September 1968 I was accompanied by Clare's successor, Jean Purdy, who shared the driving with me. Jean Purdy, a fair-haired, very English-looking young woman, was more than a laboratory technician – she had also been a nurse at one time. I soon learnt how quietly determined she was, enthused and utterly loyal. I was lucky to have Jean Purdy as an assistant. Those early mornings with Ruth coming to the front door to see us off now, in retrospect, seem nostalgically pleasant. Early mornings in Cambridge can be incredibly beautiful, and being awake and about when others are still asleep makes one feel particularly virtuous. But it was a tiring drive to Oldham, for we always had to put our foot down hard on the accelerator. We only allowed ourselves one brief stop – it was always near the Doncaster by-pass at a rather hideous transport cafe where we had a cup of stewed tea while another customer would put sixpence into the juke box. For a few minutes perhaps we would listen to a protest song – Bob Dylan or Joan Baez singing 'The Times They Are a-Changing' or 'Where Have All the Flowers Gone?' – and then we would resume our fast drive. Elsewhere there was a war in Vietnam. But we had business in Oldham, Lancashire.

Ironically, our next important step forward was taken in Cambridge, not in Oldham. One of our Ph.D students, Barry Bavister, had been trying to achieve fertilization *in vitro* of hamster eggs. After a year of attempts he had devised and refined a new culture fluid which allowed him a remarkable incidence of success. His culture fluid contained an energy source, also a few salts, a protein extracted from cow serum and penicillin. The fluid was very alkaline and it was loaded with bicarbonate.

'Since you have been so successful with hamster fertilization using that culture fluid, perhaps I could try it with human ova and spermatozoa?' I suggested.

I took some of his fluid to Oldham next time, and used it to ripen some eggs. When they were ripe, I added spermatozoa, just to see what would happen. To my delight, the next day the sperms were beginning to push through the outer membrane of the egg, and had passed through it and were lying close to the edge of three of the eggs. This was exciting. There was a possibility that fertilization was occurring. Other journeys to Oldham in October, before my lectures began again in the university, gave tantalizing suggestions of success, of those initial stages of fertilization, but I couldn't be sure because the facilities in the small room in Oldham were not good enough. I tried taking eggs from Oldham to Cambridge, strapping them to a container against my body to keep them warm during the journey, and then ripening and fertilizing them there, but they didn't appreciate the long car journey and the attempt was not very successful.

The decisive day came in March 1968. Over the telephone my old friend, Molly Rose, told me she was about to operate on a patient who would need to lose an ovary. 'So would you like some ovarian tissue?' asked Molly. I sent Jean Purdy to collect it at once. This was the last piece of ovarian tissue that I was to obtain from the Edgware General Hospital. It yielded me twelve human eggs. Those eggs were soon ripening in mixtures of the culture medium I had used over many years to which some of Barry's fluid had been added. Thirty-six hours later we judged they were ready for fertilization. There was no opportunity in Cambridge of obtaining sperms exposed to the female reproductive tract, so again we collected our own spermatozoa and, after washing them mildly and simply in a centrifuge, I added them to nine of the twelve eggs, leaving three as controls, and placing them all in Barry's culture medium. I looked at my watch. It was time for coffee.

'I'll meet you here in ten hours,' I arranged with Barry. 'Then we'll have a look and see how good your culture fluid is.' Barry Bavister, a dark-haired, humorous and amiable character, was usually very talkative, and we chatted for a while before separating.

This was now our most serious attempt at human fertilization, with everything under better organization than ever before. Fertilization had become a major bottleneck; was it just beginning to break? We had had suggestions of success in Oldham, even

though those initial laparoscopies, successfully accomplished by
Patrick, to recover spermatozoa from the Fallopian tubes, had not
led to fertilization.

The clocks in Cambridge had struck 7 p.m. when Barry and I
climbed the long flights of stairs up to my laboratory, and looked
down the microscope. I peered down first, with Barry at my side.
I held my breath. A spermatozoon was just passing into the first
egg. We examined and re-examined it and there was no doubt.
Marvellous. An hour later, we looked at the second egg. Yes,
there it was, the earliest stages of fertilization. A spermatozoon
had entered the egg without any doubt – we had done it.

'Yes,' I said softly.

Barry Bavister was impatient to have his turn and look. He,
too, was excited. We examined the other eggs and found more
and more evidence. Some ova were in the early stages of fertilization with the sperm tails following the sperm heads into the
depths of the egg; others were even more advanced with two
nuclei – one from the sperm, one from the egg – as each gamete
donated its genetic component to the embryo. I moved away
excitedly from the microscope allowing Barry to peer down.

The picture was not perfect. It seldom is when eggs are
fertilized after ripening artificially in culture rather than in the
ovary itself. But there was no question about it, none at all. All
those years of striving for this and here it was: after ten hours in
Barry's culture medium the human spermatozoa had wriggled
their way through the membrane deep into the egg.

'Your fluid's a great success,' I said.

I needed more eggs. I would repeat the procedure. Well, I
would be able to do that quite easily with Patrick's help in
Oldham. Laparoscopies would not be needed to recover spermatozoa from the female reproductive tract. That was no longer
necessary. All those manoeuvres I had carried out earlier – those
sperm-packed chambers that had been inserted into the wombs
of those North Carolina ladies – that, too, had been a waste of
endeavour and time. Once again orthodox scientific opinion had
been proved wrong. Barry Bavister, peering down through that
microscope, could also see how wrong it was.

At Oldham, using Barry's magic culture fluid, Patrick and I
now repeated the experiment. Twelve women whose ovaries had
to be removed for serious medical reasons provided us with the
necessary eggs over the next few months. We fertilized many

more eggs and were able to make detailed examinations of the successive stages of fertilization. We also took care to photograph everything now going on under the microscope because we would have to persuade colleagues of the truth of our discoveries. The fact is our chosen field of research has always been replete with fantasy. Too many in the recent past have made wild claims of achieving fertilization without offering supporting evidence, with no concept of the ripening programme, with no evidence of spermatozoa driving their way through the membranes and into the eggs, with no accompanying photographs of the two nuclei indicating successful fertilization. False claims occur because, to the inexperienced eye, degenerating eggs can resemble growing eggs. Moreover normal conceptions, normal births, can innocently be claimed as a result of an embryo transfer, for every gynaecologist knows how a woman, infertile for years, may spontaneously conceive and deliver a healthy infant. Some unknown and mysterious trigger, a change of house, the relief of some mysterious distress, some change in her metabolism, can result in a conception which hitherto the woman and all concerned had thought virtually impossible. So we needed proof irrefutable. And now we had it and intended to publish it in *Nature*. We had crossed a major hurdle. We knew our paper, our photographs, would result in an explosion of publicity – though not of such proportions as proved to be the case.

'There'll be opposition,' Patrick said. 'I just hope everybody will understand what we are trying to do and why.'

John Maddox, the newly appointed editor of *Nature*, was enthusiastic about our material. We had accumulated sufficient results from fifty-six eggs and we presented our little paper in February 1969, very objectively, in low key, in a very technical way. It made no difference – the response was intense. There were blazing headlines in the national press: 'LIFE IS CREATED IN TEST TUBE.' The telephone at home and in the laboratory at Cambridge began to ring and ring. The voices at the other end of the phone were almost all congratulatory or inquisitive.

Publicly there were those like the Archbishop of Liverpool, Dr George Beck, who cried out angrily that our experiments were 'morally wrong'. But we had our champions too. Baroness Summerskill, for example, told the press, 'This news has come on a most appropriate day. I was just reading a Valentine card.

Valentine was the saint of love – and this is all about how the
sperm can meet the ovum.' Baroness Summerskill did not
consider that ethical problems were complexly involved. 'It is
a matter of a woman who wants to be a mother and who is
unable to obtain fertilization in any other way,' she said.

What worried most commentators, though, were the implications rather than the direct consequence of 'the first successful fertilization of a human egg in a test tube', as *The
Times* called it. Their leader writer was preoccupied with the
moral problems of selective breeding, of eugenics: 'The chea-
pest and surest way for any small impoverished country to
improve its wealth and influence would be to concentrate on
breeding a race of intellectual giants. So much depends these
days on the intelligence of a nation's manpower that this
could within a generation have a dramatic effect on the
relative positions of different countries. As soon as one nation
adopted a policy of effective selective breeding, therefore,
others might well feel compelled to follow suit. The threat
that this would pose to accepted human values would be
extremely grave. There can be no slick answers to this
challenge, but it is not too soon to begin considering the
nature of the problem.'

Other newspapers, other concerns. William Breckon, the
science correspondent, was exercised about the future possibility of cloning which he felt our experiments somehow had
brought nearer: 'The test tube time-bomb is ticking away
.... Yesterday's dramatic news from Cambridge is just one
part of a tremendous explosion in the science of biology which
in the next few decades will open up even more shattering –
and frightening – possibilities .... Some of the most significant discoveries are being made in the microscopic world of
the living cell. Among them, the possibility of producing
hundreds of identical living organisms from just a single living
organism. Already scientists in Cambridge and in the USA
have had success in doing this with carrots and other vegeta-
bles. Carrot cells from a single plant can be grown in a special
broth to produce some 10,000 new growing carrots. And there
is no reason, say the scientists, why this method should not be
translated to animals and ultimately human beings. Agricul-
turalists are watching developments closely for it holds out

the promise of producing replicas of prize-winning sheep and cattle. Producing human beings in this way is obviously a long way off but leading scientists regard it as a distinct practical possibility. Ultimately we could have the know-how to breed these groups of human beings – called 'clones' after the Greek word for a throng – to produce a cohort of super-astronauts or dustmen, soldiers or senators, each with identical physical and mental characteristics most suited to do the job they have to do. Human birth without sexual contact is already a fact – with artificial insemination. The Cambridge breakthrough brings "test tube" babies a step nearer!'

I put down the newspapers and said to Ruth, 'That article by Patrick, Barry and me in *Nature* certainly stirred it up.'

'I suppose Barry Bavister must feel very pleased about it all,' Ruth remarked.

'I hope so,' I answered.

When we had looked down the microscope and observed those fertilized eggs he had been as delighted as I. Yet in some ways he had played it cool. I felt – perhaps wrongly – that he may have had some small reservations about the implications of our work. There were other scientists, though, who irritated us because they disbelieved our claims, pointing out that the entry of a spermatozoon into an egg without fertilization was a well-known phenomenon. Lord Rothschild, for instance, wrote a letter to *Nature* on 8 March 1969: 'Everyone knows that development involves the repeated division of the egg into more and more cells. No division was achieved in the experiments of Edwards *et al.* . . . ,' Rothschild thundered. 'These observations in no sense imply that I disapprove of the work: nor that I do not admire it as a preliminary experiment, although similar work has been done before . . . . Nevertheless, the claim to have fertilized a human egg outside the mother . . . . is premature. Every gametologist knows how difficult it is to be sure that a mammalian egg has been fertilized . . . . Parthogenesis and the entry of a spermatozoon into an egg without fertilization are well-known phenomena.'

I had a bit of fun answering this criticism. Lord Rothschild had recently published his own book on fertilization. His frontispiece showed a mouse egg in an earlier stage than our human eggs and he described it as undergoing fertilization.

There was a chink in his armour, not in mine. I was happy to point this out in *Nature:* 'Indeed Rothschild is hoist with his own petard, for the frontispiece to his book on fertilization shows a mouse egg with a spermatozoon in the perivitelline space and labelled, "A live fertilized mouse egg showing the whole spermatozoon in the cytoplasm". This illustration shows fertilization in the same early stage as that in our figure 4B which presents a human egg with a perivitelline spermatozoon.'

Of course we replied to all criticisms as best we could. We believed it was essential to ventilate the implications and emerging possibilities of our work so that public opinion could come into play and the law-makers debate and formulate rules of conduct for scientists and for the sake of society. Hence the interviews I gave, the increasing number of conferences I was to attend, the lectures I was to deliver whether in Washington, Delhi or Jerusalem. It was a question of prompting science and the law to move more swiftly, harmoniously, and with greater confidence, in keeping pace with advances in human embryology and other disciplines.

At this time my interest in politics revived. I joined the local Labour Party in Cambridge. But my primary preoccupation was what it had always been – to study human embryology and allow women, who were seemingly condemned for ever to a life of infertility, to bear their own children fathered by their husbands.

13
Four Beautiful Human Blastocysts

Robert Edwards

Our success in fertilizing eggs *in vitro* had been a decisive step. What we needed to do now was to take eggs that had ripened not in the culture fluid but in the ovary itself. We had to solve another major puzzle: the growth of eggs after fertilization. Problems of embryonic development seemed likely to accompany the use of human eggs that had ripened *in vitro* – all animal work confirmed that. M. C. Chang had reported how he had fertilized rabbit eggs that had ripened *in vitro* but the resulting embryos, though at first appearing normal, had soon died. My own animal research confirmed his work in rabbits, had extended it to cows, and had borne out the likelihood of abnormalities in such developing embryos.

It was a question then of Patrick obtaining the ripened eggs directly from women by laparoscopy – to withdraw eggs from the ovary without damaging them in any way. No one had ever done that before. But already I had evidence of Patrick's extraordinary surgical skill and his ability to use the laparoscope superbly.

'Yes,' said Patrick. 'If we can find a way to aspirate the eggs, laparoscopy should be invaluable for this purpose. It makes few demands on the patient, permits many manipulations in the abdominal cavity and can be used repeatedly in the same patient.'

Soon Jean and I had devised a simple, well-designed piece of apparatus that could be used at laparoscopy for the collection of eggs by sucking them gently by means of a vacuum from the little cystic-like structures, the ovarian follicles, in which they developed to maturity.

Our plans were drawn up. First, the volunteer patients would have to be given hormones to impose some control over the menstrual cycle and to stimulate the ripening of the eggs in the ovary – rather as I had done with those mice in Edinburgh a decade or so earlier. (The hormone preparations, often called fertility drugs, had improved considerably in the last few years.) Second, at a critical time, near the end of the ripening programme, Patrick would have to collect them and then I, using Barry's culture fluid, would try and fertilize these eggs with the ejaculated spermatozoa of the patient's husband.

So now we had to involve patients in our work. We had to ask Patrick's infertile patients, those desperate for help and willing to undergo many trials in the hope of one day having their own babies, to cooperate in a project that was still in its stumbling early stages. We both felt strongly that research involving women and men should only be undertaken with the greatest caution and with the greatest care – and that physical demands made upon them should be as light as possible. We both agreed that their hopes must not be raised unjustifiably and that they fully understood the situation – the opportunities and dangers and how they would be involved.

We soon discovered that patients needed to be restrained from volunteering too much. Patients would offer themselves for a second laparoscopy or even to come into Oldham General Hospital twelve times a year if necessary! One of our first patients was a dark-haired lady in her late thirties. At her bedside she said to me, 'Mr Steptoe has explained everything, exactly what is needed, and I'm glad to help all I can even if, finally, what you manage to do only becomes valuable to other women.'

We started cautiously, using low amounts of hormones to stimulate the ovary and then a touch of HCG to induce the ripening process. Fortunately I had a shrewd idea about the ripening programme, knowing it to be about thirty-six hours from all those early years of culturing human eggs. Some American workers had confirmed these results and extended them in a few patients. In the event my prediction was accurate, and soon we had a routine established. Patrick gave patients the 'fertility' hormone on the third or fourth day of their menstrual cycle, HCG on day 10 while I was in Cambridge, and performed laparoscopy thirty-two hours later. I would drive fast to Oldham, timing my arrival about thirty hours after the injection of HCG, and stay there for two or more hours after his laparoscopy, sometimes preparing the eggs for examination before immediately returning to Cambridge. Patrick's laparoscopy was fluent and I admired the dexterity with which he used his tiny instruments inside the abdomen.

Occasionally I would stay overnight at my mother's place in nearby Manchester. 'I wouldn't work as hard as you do,' Ruth would say to me, seeing me off for the umpteenth time. 'Take care how you drive.' Everybody in Cambridge knew I was travelling regularly to Oldham. Alan Parkes had now retired and Bunny Austin who had taken over from him gave me every encouragement. But it was a wearing business, driving 360 miles there and back over poor roads, sometimes after a working session or a lecture in Cambridge. It was worthwhile though, every mile of it: Patrick's ability to collect eggs from the ovary steadily improved and I saw the ripening eggs precisely ready for fertilization as they were withdrawn from the ovary.

Within a month or two we observed once again all the stages of fertilization. I called over Patrick from the clinic to the laboratory so that he could observe what Jean Purdy and I had already looked at: how only *one* spermatozoon had penetrated each egg. This was important because if more than one sperm had entered the ovum chromosomal imbalance would occur – triploidy or worse. While we were waiting for Patrick I recalled how last October he had been excited when he had witnessed in this very lab our first fertilization. 'A fertilized human egg!' he had said. 'I am one of the three or four people in the world who has genuinely seen this phenomenon and it's taking place in Oldham.' But now the eggs had ripened inside their mother, not in our culture fluids, and were full of the promises of natural growth.

We were poised for the earliest period of human embryo growth – that period when the round fertilized one-cell egg divides after a day or two, beautifully and cleanly, into two equal-sized cells, then into four cells, eight cells, and so on. If he were ever to witness that, Patrick could stick out his chest further – because even fewer people had witnessed human life at such an early stage. The available knowledge of the few-days-old fertilized ovum was scanty indeed.

I was suggesting to Jean that we should modify Barry's culture fluid and try to bring it into accord with the natural conditions pertaining to the human body, when Patrick arrived.

He moved towards the microscope. 'Success again,' I said. But I was thinking much more about the next stage – the cell divisions of the fertilized ovum, the cleaving of the embryo. Then Jean and I would have to remain at Oldham General for days on end. Already I had to leave the family on their own too often. Ruth was very supportive but I knew she would miss me as much as I missed her. 'Wonderful,' I heard Patrick say as he peered down the microscope. 'Beautiful and fascinating.'

Everything was now set for the growth of the embryos. Here again was a possible hurdle that could take years to overcome. It was well known at that time that the embryos of some species grew well in culture, such as those of the rabbit, whereas others were very difficult indeed. For some reason or other, embryos of several animals faced a block in culture just after they had started growing, usually around the two-cell stage; even today this problem has not been fully solved in several animal species including rats, mice, hamsters and others. The rabbit enjoyed the reputation of being a good embryo to grow, and also of being a good mother to support the embryos of other species; cow and sheep eggs will grow happily within the rabbit, and can even be flown around the world within it to establish herds in distant countries. We transferred some fertilized human eggs into rabbits to see if they would also grow there, but they didn't. This brief episode with rabbits led to all sorts of rumours in the press and elsewhere, and to a description of me taking hundreds of embryos to Cambridge, and of Patrick driving his Mercedes through Oldham with a rabbit in the seat next to him!

We had to test the fertilized human eggs in several different culture solutions to find which was the best for their growth. We first tried out simple solutions that had been designed for mouse embryos. The number of human eggs available was limited – one or two from each patient – and only two or three patients a month. So our commuting to Oldham was irregular and infrequent even though we had to stay over for longer periods.

To my delight our rare human eggs began their development satisfactorily in the 'mouse' culture fluid. One day after fertilization the human ovum divided into two cells and in two to three days into four cells. To observe a living, vibrant embryo beginning its early steps of development is a most stimulating sight for an embryologist – whether it be mouse, rabbit, sea-urchin or human.

None of the embryos developed further than eight cells. So we changed the culture fluid. Finally the one we chose had been prepared by an American – his fluid was called Ham's F10. A touch of serum from the patients themselves, we discovered, was also needed. So, in this complex fluid stuffed full of vitamins, amino acids, fats and sugars – all the nutrients required to cover the remotest needs of tissues destined to become those of a human being – the embryos thrived.

The beginnings of life have never failed to fascinate me. It is a period rich and strange in change and movement. The microscopic embryonic cells move elegantly and precisely along their appointed pathway, forming a succession of shapes before they emerge into the pattern of their human form. I was thrilled when I observed the embryos we had incubated divide into two cells, four cells, eight cells and more, each cell with its own nucleus. Nor was there any sign of damage or fragmentation. There was every indication of normality. I am still thrilled as an egg divides and develops for, in addition to the beauty of its growth the embryo is passing through a critical period of life of great exploration: it becomes magnificently organized, switching on its own biochemistry, increasing in size, and preparing itself quickly for implantation in the womb. After that its organs form – the cells gradually become capable of development into heart, lung, brain, eye. What a unique and wonderful process it is, as the increasing number of cells diverge and specialize in a delicate, integrated and coordinated manner. One day all the secrets of this early development may be known and those same secrets may help us to repair the ravages and defects in the tissues of sick and ageing men and women.

Returning to Cambridge in the car we had rented, both Jean and I were silent most of the journey. Then half way home I found myself saying out loud: 'These early stages of growth – they include so many fundamentals. The movement of chromosomes in the egg – a single small mistake can lead to Mongolism or some other chromosomal error. The early embryo is in a period of life when inheritance can be modified before its relatively few cells are committed for ever to their fate in the body. You know, the succession of events – fertilization, the cleavage of the embryo, its implantation, can each be manipulated for purposes of contraception . . . .' We were close to Doncaster and that transport café. I took my foot off the accelerator, and soon we were parking the car.

At Oldham we now moved confidently forward. Every embryo was precious and we improved our methods of obtaining them by gradually increasing the amount of hormone injected into Patrick's patients. We also moved to a more convenient room. Though it had earlier been used for storing soiled linen and for laundry it did have the advantage of being next to the operating theatre and being under the keen and dedicated eye of Patrick Steptoe's senior operating nurse, Muriel Harris. There we continued to observe those cleaving embryos, sadly having to flatten them in order to examine their nuclei and chromosomes under the microscope. This was a heartbreaking procedure considering all the efforts we had made to obtain and nurture them. But it had to be done to make sure they were growing normally. Once again we wrote our results up and sent them for publication in *Nature*.

We were now ready to let some eight-celled embryos continue their development further instead of flattening them for microscopic examination. It would probably take five days to reach the stage called a blastocyst. This is the last stage of growth before the embryo begins its implantation in the mother's womb. We reached this target of trying for the blastocyst more rapidly than I had anticipated. Patrick was collecting eggs from the ovary with a high rate of success and we were fertilizing them and supporting their cleavage. Within twelve months of achieving fertilization we had enough spare embryos to consider undertaking this final step towards the blastocyst. It meant a prolonged stay in Oldham, arriving before Patrick's laparoscopy, achieving fertilization and cleavage, and awaiting the next several days of growth.

'In all it's a week's commitment,' I said. 'There's my work at Cambridge – not to mention the gentle demands of my family.'

'Perhaps we could share the waiting game,' suggested Jean. 'That way neither of us will be too long away from Cambridge.'

So sometimes I remained in Oldham while she returned to Cambridge. It was like a relay race. For then she would drive north and relieve me after a day or two. It was a hell of a schedule, but events were moving forward, forward, steadily forward, and we did not wish to interrupt our flow of work. All of us – Patrick, Jean, myself – knew that soon, under the microscope, we might well see the major modifications in the structure and shape of the three-to-four days fertilized embryo as it established its axis – where the head would grow, where the body form – as it prepared itself for implantation in the womb.

One afternoon Jean was on sentry-guard watching over some four-day-old embryos and I was attending to my university duties in Cambridge. Jean called on the telephone. 'It looks promising,' she said and described what she had seen. I asked her if I should come up. 'I'll phone you tomorrow if there's any further change,' she said.

The next evening after dinner the telephone rang again. This time at my home. Again Jean's voice in the receiver but now it was really excited. 'Something is happening,' she said. 'Things I've not seen before. You must come up.'

It seemed the cells had pushed and shoved their way in their appointed directions, fluid had accumulated within the embryo – first in small secretions between the cells, then later it had run together to form a large confluent pool at its centre. A group of cells, thin and transparent, formed on the surface of the embryo as it literally turned into a sphere filled with liquid.

'Not one expanding embryo but four of them,' cried Jean excitedly.

Her descriptions of the embryos were so exciting that I had to journey to Oldham immediately. I had a rented car waiting – in those days we always seemed to have a rented car waiting. 'I'll be with you as soon as I can,' I said.

Ruth had overheard my conversation and had gone upstairs to put some things in an overnight bag for me. I looked at my watch. It was after eight. If I left right away I would be in Oldham by eleven o'clock. 'Make sure you stop and rest at least once on the way,' Ruth advised. I kissed her, then made for the car.

I drove through the night. The roads were reasonably empty; occasional lights of oncoming cars; then darkness apart from my own headlights picking up the phosphorescent cat's-eyes. I kept thinking – *was this it, at last?* Waiting for me in Oldham *would there be normal blastocysts?* I was too impatient to stop at that transport café near the Doncaster by-pass. I was glad there were no police cars on the look-out for motorists speeding that night, otherwise I would have been booked. I think I must have touched ninety miles an hour – the car would not go faster.

Arriving in Oldham I went immediately to our small laboratory next to the operating theatre. It was a tiny room, six feet by
nine feet. I opened the door and Jean, who was waiting, turned
towards me. She placed the embryos under the microscope and I
looked down the lens. It was an unbelievable sight: four beautiful
human blastocysts, round spheres of cells filled with fluid, with
their two types of cell – one thin and delicate, on the surface of
each sphere, destined to turn into the placenta, which would
nourish the foetus throughout the nine months' gestation; the
other a beautiful disc of foetal cells, the beginning of the foetus
as it started its journey towards life. Light, transparent, floating,
expanding slightly, but still smaller than a pinpoint: there they
were, four excellent blastocysts. The intrinsic beauty of it!

I knew that instant that we had reached our goal: the early
stages of human life were all there in our culture fluids, just as
we wanted. Our target had been reached far quicker than anyone
expected, including ourselves – and even as I gazed down at those
embryos, wondering what to do with them, there was no doubt
in my mind that the whole field was now wide open. This was
the moment when everything became possible, when my hopes
and endeavours over a long time began to take on their final
realization. And all this within two years of teaming up with
Patrick. These embryos had developed well past the stage where
they could be replaced in the mother's uterus. Indeed, those four
blastocysts could have been used for that purpose. But, no, we
could not do that – conditions in the tiny laboratory were not
good enough. There was no sterile, filtered air, no clean surfaces
or other essentials in this tiny annexe to the operating theatre.
We did not know whether they had normal nuclei or chromosomes. The time was not ripe to replant them into their mothers.
Reluctantly we would have to prepare these embryos for examination. We would have to flatten them on glass slides to look at
their nuclei and chromosomes.

We had a feeling of being greatly privileged to see those
human blastocysts. All we had done was to set up the right
conditions for them to grow, and we had then been able to
witness some of the wonderful events of embryology, events
occurring every day many times over within many women. Like
so many discoveries in science, the realization of an objective, of
a goal, which clinches and clarifies years of effort makes one
more humble, more aware of the wonders of Nature as they

unfold in all their beauty. We had merely observed them, nothing more; someone else designed them.

Suddenly, I felt tired. All in. It was time to drive over to my mother's house in Manchester. I looked at my watch. She would be asleep by now but I had the key to the door. We decided to leave the blastocysts overnight to grow a little more and to show Patrick them next morning.

'See you in the morning, Jean,' I said, as she went to the Nurses' Home over the road. I strode out to the car park, which was situated between the hospital wing where we now worked and the pathology laboratory where we used to be. As I walked to the car, I looked up at all the stars, the moon, the night sky over Oldham, and considered the equally amazing sights I had just seen under my microscope.

14

The Wounds of Opposition

Robert Edwards

Next morning the temptation to replace the blastocysts into the mother on the spot was very strong, and I have often wondered what might have happened had we succumbed. They belonged not to us but to the wife and husband who had donated their eggs and spermatozoa.

'What are we going to do with them?' asked Patrick.

'We're going to flatten them for chromosomes,' I replied.

'What do I tell my patients?' Patrick persisted.

Patrick knew, as I did, that there would always be some embryos that would not be replaced in their mothers. Instead they would have to be examined, they would have to be fixed and stained for microscopic examination and, as a result, their growth ended. Was it justifiable to use these blastocysts so that we could investigate early human growth? Did they have any rights? Society at large appears to allow them rights, not at fertilization, but later in pregnancy. The intrauterine devices of contraception that some women wear ensure that any cleaving embryos are expelled and lost naturally without anyone even being aware of them. Indeed, abortion laws remove the right to life from much older foetuses, including those with inherited defects at three to four months of gestation if their handicap is too great to be accepted by their parents. The embryos cleaving in our culture fluids were minute and immature without the vestige of an organ or even a tissue compared with those aborted under the law.

Of course, absolutists disagree. They regard fertilization as a kind of holy event above the interference of man. The overwhelming consensus of society and its laws, as well as many observations in biology, do not sustain the absolutist point of view about fertilization as the essential step that instantly confers

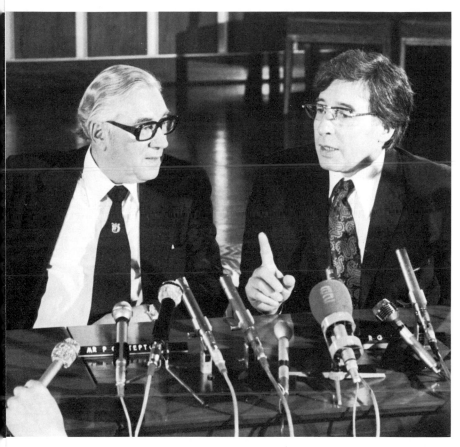

Patrick Steptoe, FRCS, FRCOG (*left*) and Robert Edwards, DSc, PhD, at the press conference in Oldham announcing the birth of the world's first 'test tube' baby. [*Daily Telegraph*]

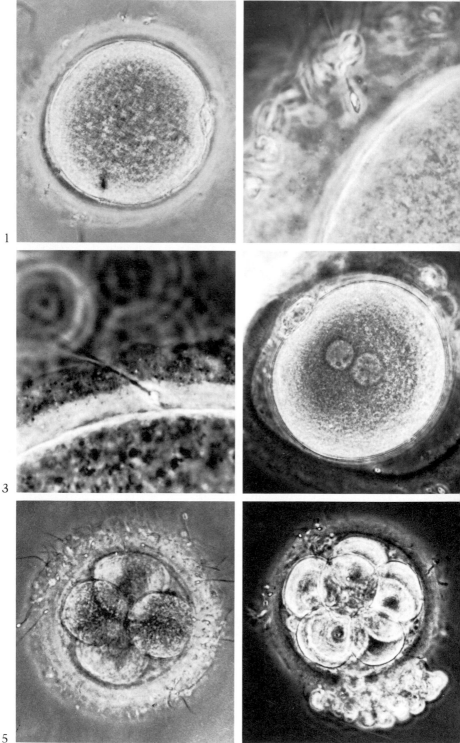

1

3

5

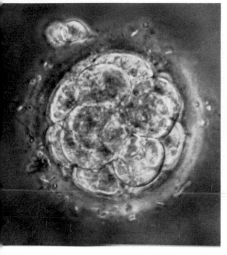
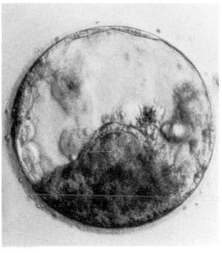

THE BEGINNING OF LIFE
Ovulation, fertilization and cleavage of the human egg

This remarkable series of photographs taken under the microscope shows the various stages of development from the fertilisation of the human egg to formation of the embryo.

1. The egg, taken from an ovary, has been ripened. Round the circumference are membranes (seen as a hazy substance) which the sperms, clearly visible, are trying to penetrate.

2. One spermatozoon is penetrating the membrane –

3. – and has now reached the surface of the egg. This is the first dramatic meeting between the sperm and the egg.

4. About eight hours later, two pro-nuclei are observed, the larger formed by the sperm and the smaller by egg chromosomes. These will form a single cell which will divide into two cells and then –

5. – into four cells. Spermatozoa which have been prevented from entering can still be seen outside the membrane.

6. The four cells have each divided again. It was at this stage (eight-cell) that Steptoe replaced the fertilised egg in Lesley Brown's womb. Attached to the embryo can be seen the radiating crown which assists in the secretion of nourishing bio-chemical fluids.

7. A sixteen-cell human embryo. This is the stage when the egg was replaced in Mrs Montgomery's womb.

8. The blastocyst. The fertile egg is now complete with all its cells. The dark portion known as the embryonic disc will become the foetus (see drawing on page 132). Within the sphere there is fluid surrounded by cells which will become the placenta.

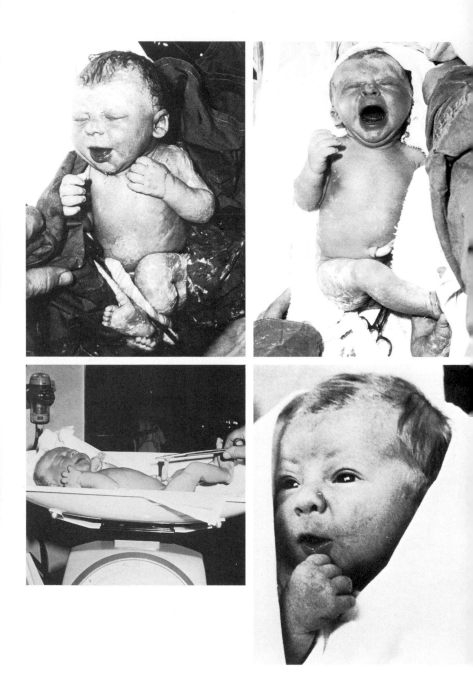

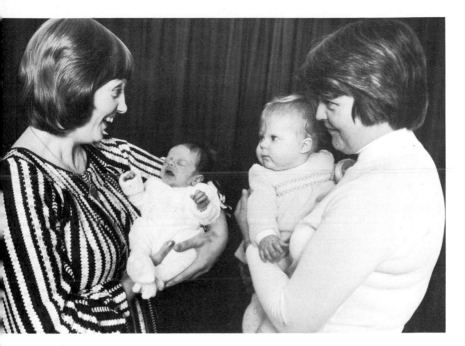

Facing page: Louise Joy Brown, the world's first 'test tube' baby, aged 30 seconds (*top left*), 5 minutes (*top right*), 10 minutes (*bottom left*), and one day

Above: Two happy mothers with babies which they had been told they could never have – Grace Montgomery and Alastair (*left*), Lesley Brown and Louise. [*Associated Newspapers*]

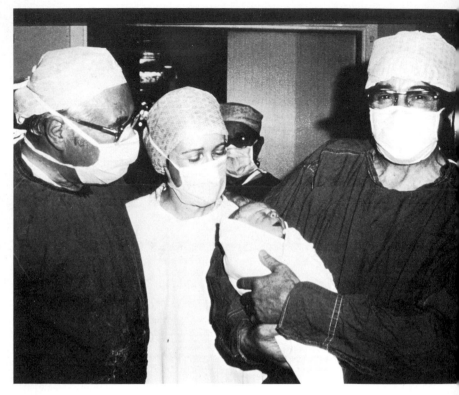

After ten years of experiment and research, the doctor (Patrick Steptoe, *left*) and the scientist (Robert Edwards) stand with Jean Purdy, the technical assistant, holding the first baby ever to be conceived outside the mother's womb. This photograph was taken immediately after the completion of the Caesarean operation.

on the fertilized cell the full rights of the individual. As a matter of fact, life is highly organized in the egg before fertilization and an embryo can develop to advanced stages of growth by being stimulated artificially by that process called parthenogenesis. A single blastocyst is not the pinpoint of one life necessarily: it will on occasion divide to produce two, three, four or even five identical offspring, each capable of normal life. Fertilization is for me but one step on the long road to birth. And there are many other fundamental steps on the way.

'What do I tell my patients?' Patrick had asked.

'I've got to see that the cell nuclei and the chromosomes are good,' I had replied. 'You'll be able to explain to them that we've taken another step forward.'

This was dramatically true – the growth of the blastocysts suggested wonderful new opportunities in science and medicine. And when we examined the blastocysts, finding no signs of aberrant development, it became abundantly clear that we now needed better facilities, better equipment, better microscopes, better measuring devices, a sterile laboratory.

For the time being we could perfect our methods, produce more embryos and examine their chromosomes. We had to know whether their state of growth was satisfactory and when exactly would be the best time in their development to replant them in their mothers. But what about that sterile laboratory?

'There's Dr Kershaw's Cottage Hospital in nearby Royton,' Patrick suggested. 'It has a small operating theatre, small and large wards and several other tiny rooms. It will cost a lot of money though to get it to the standards we require.'

'If only we could both work in Cambridge,' I said.

The years of constant travelling to Oldham were now beginning to take their toll. The days of sojourn in Lancashire played havoc with my family life. All too often I would see Ruth's face cloud over as I had to disappoint the children over some matter or as I had to cancel a party, a theatre outing, a dinner, at the last moment, while I hired a car and dashed northwards complete with equipment and necessities. Jean also had to face similar problems. It was difficult to make firm engagements with friends and relatives when there was a possibility that one late evening or at crack of dawn we would have to drive north to Patrick, who would have a patient ready. I always remember returning home on one occasion after a prolonged stay at Oldham and being surprised to discover not only new neighbours in the street but fresh colleagues in the laboratory at Cambridge. I had forgotten any previous hints of impending changes.

But a move to Cambridge would be difficult for Patrick. He was a senior and respected gynaecologist in Oldham, and he would have to leave his patients and his home to move to a new house, a new city, a new practice. Besides, there was an abundance of gynaecologists at Cambridge and the university did not have a clinical school at that time. Thus there was no possibility of a university position for him.

'On the other hand, Newmarket General Hospital is only fifteen miles away from Cambridge,' I said. 'Would you be prepared to work there?'

'Yes. I would accept a consultant post in Newmarket if that could be managed,' agreed Patrick.

To travel only fifteen miles instead of the journey to Oldham! Why, that would be wonderful. So I spoke to the Dean of Medicine in Cambridge, I gained the support of several professors, consultants, administrators and others. There was one organization in Britain that could underwrite this move – the Medical Research Council. They had the power and the influence and the financial backing to organize support for a consultant, to provide facilities and equipment.

Many months before we even submitted our proposals to the Medical Research Council our activities at Oldham were suddenly put under a floodlit lens in a most magnified and distorted fashion. It all began with an innocent enough call from a BBC producer. 'Can I come to see you?' he asked. 'We're going to do a programme about fertilization and other matters.'

'OK,' I said. 'We'll discuss it.'

I had learnt not to say too much on the telephone by now. That was one lesson Alan Parkes taught me. When the BBC producer did come to see me I backed away as fast as I could. For when I asked him, 'What will the programme be about specifically?' he replied, 'Why, about the increasing control over early life. We are going to describe things like cloning and hybrids between species – mixture of cells between species, a fusion of two different species. We'll focus on the cell fusion they are attempting at Oxford between human and mouse cells.'

'I'm not interested in participating in such a programme,' I responded sharply. 'This has got nothing to do with me.'

It all sounded sensational, science-fiction stuff. I did not want to know.

'I'm going to Oxford to see Professor Harris who's working on cell fusion. And I'll see others . . . .,' he continued.

But I declined to collaborate. He seemed far from happy with my response. His voice changed. There was a sense of bared knuckles as he took his leave and said, 'If you don't come on the programme voluntarily I'll involve you in one way or another.'

'Goodbye,' I said.

I did not ponder on the threatening posture of that BBC producer. I had other preoccupations. Scientists were visiting me from abroad. I had become involved in local Labour Party politics. Christmas was coming, presents to buy, cards to be sent off. That winter I hardly drove up to Oldham. There was still confirmatory work to be undertaken but for the moment there was no urgency. Jean, too, was glad of the respite in our constant travelling to Lancashire.

I remembered sitting at home with Ruth one evening and watching the BBC programme that I had declined to participate in. At once I was glad my response had been negative, because the programme opened with a picture of the atom bomb explosion in Hiroshima and an accompanying innuendo that scientific work led to such catastrophic conclusions. Then we were offered a view of my laboratory windows at Cambridge while a sepul-chral voice intoned over, 'It's only a few hundred paces down the road from this laboratory that Rutherford split the atom – and we all know what that led to.'

'Good job they don't know our relationship to Rutherford,' Ruth remarked.

The sepulchral voice then quoted, out of context, some of my more dramatic remarks about growing human embryos in the lab. Subsequently there were sequences from Oxford about cell fusion and cloning.

When the programme ended I switched off the television set and said, 'Well, I'm glad I never gave them a direct quote.'

Terrible Brave-New-World visions such as those we had just viewed irritated me. They still do. They are based on the pessimistic assumption that the worst will happen. The whole edifice of their argument is fragile – that nuclear physics led inevitably to the atom bomb, electricity to the electric chair, civil engineering to the gas-chambers. Surely acceptance of the beginning does not necessitate embracing undesirable ends?

Even well-meant attempts to describe our work were unsuccessful. Sometimes spectacularly so. When asked by a producer in February 1970, Patrick decided to collaborate in making a television film on our work for *Horizon*, and organized their visit, complete with cameras, to his operating theatre. He wanted to provide films of the laparoscopy, showing the ovary and the womb, and how it was all done, with one or two questions to a typical patient, who would remain anonymous.

It did not work out that way. Somehow or other, the TV crew got to the patient's home for a full-scale interview with full personal details and photographs, and everything duly appeared on the programme. I was in India at the time, and was astonished to be approached by reporters describing our patient and her interview. What Patrick went through back home I can hardly imagine.

On 24 February, the day after the programme, the newspapers were full of front page headlines: 'WIFE IS WAITING FOR A TEST-TUBE BABY' (*Daily Mirror*); 'COUPLE PLAN TEST-TUBE BABY' (*Daily Express*); 'WIFE WHO HOPES FOR A TEST-TUBE BABY' (*Daily Sketch*); 'DOCTORS START BABY OUTSIDE THE WOMB' (*The Guardian*). What the newspapers concentrated on was the Oldham patient. Some spoke of her as being 'the guinea-pig mother of the test-tube era'. Immediately other scientists and doctors were interviewed and their instant comments printed, so that on Wednesday, the 25th, the newspapers still led with the story: BABIES STORM GROWING (*Daily Express*); TEST TUBE BABIES RAISE MORAL ISSUE (*Daily Telegraph*); MOVE TO THRESHOLD OF GENETIC ENGINEERING (*The Times*); BAN THE TEST TUBE BABY (*Sun*).

Everybody seemed to comment on our work. Dr Derek Stevenson, secretary of the British Medical Association, said that, like organ transplantation, fertilization *in vitro* carried with it difficult ethical problems that called for careful thought by doctors and others; the Church of England Information Office said that the development would need careful assessment on moral, social and legal grounds; Father John McDonald, a former Professor of Moral Theology, said the marriage contract did not give marriage partners the right to children but the right to natural sexual intercourse from which children might result. Another point which he felt

Catholics would have further objections to was the way in which the husband's semen was obtained. Dr Douglas Bevis of Sheffield Jessop Hospital, who was reported to have been doing 'test-tube' baby research for eighteen months, declared that the publicity would give false hope to thousands of childless couples and that it was wrong to claim test-tube babies could be produced because many major difficulties still had to be overcome.

Mr Norman St John Stevas, the Conservative Member of Parliament who had opposed the Abortion Bill, said that he thought 'test-tube' babies would be legitimate in cases where the woman's own egg was used, fertilized by her own husband's semen and where it was impossible for her to have a baby in any other way. As for our patient who had been sought out and grilled by scores of reporters, she merely said, 'I just want an ordinary healthy baby after all this time. If what I am doing will give heart to childless wives throughout the world then I will be even happier. I myself can't wait. There is no other hope.'

A year earlier we had experienced publicity enough when we had reported our successful fertilization *in vitro*. But the publicity and controversy following the TV programme was more intense, more intrusive. The volume of comment on our work was turned up horrendously loud. Worse, some reporters were highly irresponsible. They sought out and chased our patients in Oldham hoping to discover and interview other mothers-to-be of 'test-tube' babies. In June 1970 I happily attended a BMA meeting that discussed the relationship between doctors and the press, doctors and television. I made pungent comments, I related my experiences.

I did not shrink from any discussion related to our work in whatever context and whatever continent. These conferences on ethics and the future possibilities of medical advance became more and more common, and I participated in them even more frequently now that controversy continued increasingly and on a massive international scale. I had no doubts about the morals and ethics of our work. I accepted the right of our patients to found their family, to have their own children. I was blessed, Patrick was blessed, some of our most stringent critics were fortunate to have children of their own. It was a priceless asset. It was a gift, the relationship of parent to a developing human being. And almost within our grasp was the possibility of passing on this gift to couples who had suffered years of childlessness and frustration – who longed for children, who had indeed, as often as not, repeatedly undergone unsuccessful gynaecological operations in order to try to have children. The Declaration of Human Rights made by the United Nations includes the right to establish a family.

There were those who argued, 'Why should infertility be cured when orphans and other children are desperately awaiting adoption?' Adoption is an excellent institution but the argument implies the withdrawal of medical care from one group of people in order to solve the problems of another. Besides, many of our patients had tried to adopt children repeatedly and without success. Moreover adoption is likely to become even more difficult in the future with the spread of contraception and abortion, and with the rapid decline in the number of unwanted children. More and more couples would surely be pleading for the right to have their own child.

Others were fearful that the so-called 'test-tube' babies would be abnormal in some way.

'The next real problem,' the *New Scientist* leader-writer declared, contemplating our work, 'comes in re-introducing the blastula to the womb of the woman. The timing of this process is absolutely crucial . . . . Only one other real doubt remains. This concerns the possibility of abnormal development of the implanted human egg *in vitro*. Steptoe appears confident that abnormalities will not occur but it is rather difficult to see the reason for his optimism . . . .'

There were many prominent people whose views were resonant with this statement. But I had few fears. All my knowledge of mice, rats, rabbits, farm animals, convinced me their development would be as normal as those beginning life within their mother. The cleaving embryos are very small but very resistant to damage. They have the innate capacity to reorder and reform, to overcome the effects of drugs, X rays, and other seemingly noxious agents that scientists have exposed them to. When they cannot resist certain stimuli the embryos die – they grow normally or they succumb. There are no intermediates.

Pieces have been excised from animal embryos, they have been dissected and disaggregated into small pieces – even into single cells – then, like Humpty Dumpty, put back together again. The survivors have remained refreshingly normal, adaptable. Their powers of regeneration are astonishing. I knew this well and I told others that resistance to injury is a property of the earliest stages of embryonic life, that this resistance lasts to the blastocyst stage and perhaps further, before fading *after* the embryos become implanted in the womb to begin their formative stages of growth. It is only then that they become sensitive to noxious agents – to drugs, to X rays, traumatic shocks. It is only then that their growth may become distorted to cause physiological and mental defects in the baby. These disasters occur after the embryo has been implanted in its mother and not before, so they would not arise in our culture fluids. That was the reason, the golden rule, for Patrick's optimism. We were free of such worries provided the mother was careful once her embryo had been replaced within her.

There was only one possible exception to that golden rule: a slight error in the ripening process of the egg, a small difficulty in fertilization, a tiny failure as the embryo began to grow could result in chromosome disasters for the foetus. A small extra chromosome could gain access to the egg, coming from the mother or father, to play havoc with normal growth. It could result in Mongolism or intersexuality. And, if the eggs ripened badly, or if two spermatozoa pushed their way into one ovum, some embryos could even be triploid with 69 chromosomes.

Yes, chromosomes could be a problem but it was one that had to be kept in perspective. Most foetuses with extra chromosomes die in the womb and abort spontaneously. There is nothing novel about chromosomal upset. The number of human embryos conceived normally which begin life handicapped in this way is staggering. Almost one quarter of women who become pregnant lose their babies in the first three months because of those chromosomal discrepancies. Early human growth is littered with such failures.

No one knows why. Perhaps the chromosomal disasters occur because there is too long a delay between ovulation and intercourse – the egg having to wait until the spermatozoa arrive. These frequent chromosomal complications are unique to man. In animals such as mice, rats and rabbits, mating

occurs at oestrus, close to ovulation and so a delay in fertilization is avoided, and so also such a frequency of chromosomal
abnormality.

In any event, we had a well-proven line of defence, because
a faulty embryo implanted in its mother can be detected at
three to four months of gestation. Many thousands of foetuses
are now examined by removing a small amount of fluid
around them as they lie in the womb. This test is carried out
in order to discover disorders in the number or type of
chromosomes or some anomalies in body growth. If a defect is
found then the parents may be faced with an agonizing
decision – to abort their foetus or to allow it to survive and
develop into a subnormal baby. There are couples who,
because of their own disordered chromosomes or genes, know
that one day they will have to face up to such a choice. They
know this even before the baby is conceived. Our patients
would be in a similar situation. After all their long waiting,
after all their efforts to establish pregnancy, in the unlikely
event of that test proving a chromosomal discrepancy, their
predicament would be sad indeed. But it would be the same
predicament as others had and have to face.

Fortunately all the work that we carried out at Oldham,
while we were waiting for the Medical Research Council to
respond to our submission, confirmed that there was no cause
for worrying about chromosomal upsets. Long ago, when a
student, I had wondered, why does only one spermatozoon
enter an ovum? Years later I learnt the reason for this: once
the ovum had become fertilized a chemical change in the
membranes of the egg takes place preventing entries by other
sperms. But it crossed my mind now that the artificial conditions pertaining in the laboratory might, in some mysterious
way, interfere with this chemical alteration in the egg membranes. Supposing they remained permeable? More spermatozoa were active close to the ovum in our cultures than there
were naturally in the oviduct. That alone, perhaps, would
allow a greater likelihood of a second sperm to enter the egg.
However, the more we repeated our work at Oldham the more
confident I became that these shadowy fears of mine were
groundless.

As usual, after working at Oldham, I would stay at night
with my mother in Manchester. She was now in her seventies

and living alone – my father died in 1964. Like so many other friends and relatives she had read about our activities. Sometimes she gently asked me about it. I would explain to her how much opposition we were experiencing, sometimes even from colleagues, and how we needed more expensive facilities, preferably near Cambridge, so that our aspirations could become concrete facts. She would listen a little, then say, 'Do what's right, Bob.'

And that is what I intended to do. To carry on towards our goal, however difficult the course and whatever wounding misunderstandings arose as we travelled that course. On one occasion, at my mother's house, I talked to my elder brother, Sam, who had been reading news of our work. 'What's all this I hear about cloning or whatever it's called?' he asked me.

The popular interest in cloning is amazing. Though it is irrelevant to our work I have had to face arguments about it since our earliest days. Cloning has been effected in a few amphibians by inserting a nucleus from the cell of an adult into an unfertilized egg. It is a valuable method for animal rather than human embryology.

'We call it "clowning" not cloning,' I told Sam. 'For if it became technically possible children would suffer the gratuitous imposition of inherited characteristics. These would mimic, perhaps, a conceited and self-important donor. Should cloning ever happen the child would develop normally, be very well looked after, and have a relationship with its donor somewhat similar to that of an identical twin separated by many years of age. A curious existence but not an impossible one.'

I changed the subject and told him how, lately, I had become more involved in local politics in Cambridge. It was no longer a question of arguing solely about medical ethics. I felt strongly about the housing shortage, about the unfairness of our education system, about the inequality of opportunity among different classes. There was the repugnant war in Vietnam. There was not much an individual could do but it was no accident that I was seeing more of my colleagues in the Newnham Ward of the Labour Party.

But, returned to Cambridge, I was suddenly jolted back to my primary preoccupation. I felt a metaphorical blow when I read a scary paper that my friend Chang had published in the USA. He reported that one-half of his rats, born as a result of fertilization *in vitro*, had extremely small eyes. This puzzled and, for the moment, worried me. Was this substance for those who argued the possibility of abnormal development in the implanted human egg fertilized *in vitro*? Then, relieved, I realized that an incidence of exactly one-half of the rats owning small eyes suggested the effect of a gene carried within the rats themselves – just as Mendel had originally conjectured in his early studies. When I checked with Chang I was happy to learn that he had already discovered the gene and that, indeed, all offspring had normal eyes when he used another stock of rats for fertilization *in vitro*.

A more enduring blow was in store for us. One morning in late April 1971 I opened a letter at the Physiological Laboratory in Downing Street, Cambridge. It was from the Medical Research Council. I read:

'Dear Dr Edwards,

'The Council have now had an opportunity of considering your application made jointly with Mr P. C. Steptoe for long-term support for a programme of research in the field of human reproduction on which the advice of the Clinical Research Board and of external referees had been sought.

'I am sorry to have to tell you that, after the most careful consideration, the Council came to the conclusion that they could not agree to your request for long-term support since they had serious doubts about ethical aspects of the proposed investigations in humans, especially those relating to the implantation in women of oocytes fertilized *in vitro*, which were considered premature in view of the lack of preliminary studies on primates and the present deficiency of detailed knowledge of the possible hazards involved. Reservations were also expressed about the justifiability of employing the procedure of laparoscopy for purely experimental purposes. The application was accordingly declined.

'I realize that you will be disappointed by this news. However the Council asked that you should be told that they would be prepared to consider an application from you for support of an experimental programme of work of the type you have already proposed to be carried out in primates. Such an application would of course have to be considered *de novo* by the Council who cannot commit themselves to the provision of support . . . .'

I felt sick reading that letter. This opposition was wounding. I read it again and felt angry. I would phone Patrick. He would be amazed by their remarks, especially those about laparoscopy? Who were these external referees who pronounced on laparoscopy? Patrick had established the method in the UK and was now perhaps the leading laparoscopist in the world. Did they not know the method was quick, neat and efficient? The Council did not seem to understand fully what we had done and what we were trying to do. As for suggesting that we should work on primates, that was not possible. The fertility drugs we used successfully with our patients did not activate female monkeys very well. Accordingly, there were few, if any, ripening monkey eggs to be had, and they could not be fertilized *in vitro*, a situation still existing today.

I picked up the telephone and dialled Patrick's number. I could not accept what the MRC were saying to us. 'Serious doubts about the ethical aspects' of our work. Hell – whom did we have to convince? The telephone clicked and I heard Patrick's voice saying, 'Steptoe here.'

'I have bad news, Patrick,' I said.

Some years later, I found out that the Medical Research Council had probably been misadvised about fertilization *in vitro* and were unaware of the true situation regarding those rats with small eyes. I did not know if Chang publicly corrected his work on these rats but I certainly did in my own papers. They had obviously not been read by our critics.

15
The Shindy in Washington

Robert Edwards

The value of first testing our work on rhesus monkeys was most questionable. Monkeys might be a good model for studying the damaging effects of drugs on growing foetuses. But their earliest growth and implantation differ a great deal from human beings, and mice are a closer parallel to man. Indeed, monkeys have other disadvantages. The entrance to the womb is highly convoluted, and replanting monkey embryos would be difficult. They carry nasty viruses that could infect man. What was the point of experimenting for years and years on monkeys when they didn't respond to hormones and when the resultant outcome probably would not be relevant anyway?

Patrick and I decided to respond to the Medical Research Council's devastating refusal by drawing attention to facts such as these. On 11 June, we dictated a letter to the Council: 'Mr Chairman and Gentlemen,' we began, 'we regret your decision not to support our proposed scientific and clinical research in Cambridge .... We find the statement about the hazards of transferring embryos difficult to accept .... More than three thousand laparoscopies have been carried out in the Oldham General Hospital, with no mortality and with only occasional minor complications .... We could not perform some of the manipulations on these [primate] species which we would have to carry out on our patients .... We regret that an application for a joint scientific and medical programme of such considerable scope was rejected on the ethical grounds stated without having had an opportunity to answer the criticisms raised, and especially since there is obviously widespread scientific and medical support for our work.'

It was a sharp letter. Soon, we received an equally sharp letter back. It concluded with, ' ... I think you should know that

Council are not prepared to reconsider applications for support which they have declined, unless it can be shown either that there are certain vital new facts which might have caused them to arrive at a different decision had they known of them when the application was considered; or that there have since been changes in circumstances which might cause them to alter that decision. I can find evidence of neither of these circumstances in your letter . . . .'

There was no point in attempting to combat the Council. If I did it would be like deliberately choosing to become a character fit for a Kafka novel. Our hoped-for laboratory base at or close to Cambridge had fallen into a hole in the ground for ever. It was a great setback. We would have to continue somehow in Oldham, perhaps at that Kershaw's Cottage Hospital Patrick recommended and which he had made tentative soundings about already. But finance would be needed for Kershaw's too. We had our patients to consider. They were totally aware of the medical situation and of what we were trying to do. We had explained everything to them and they understood. Several of them were women doctors, doctors' wives, or nurses, well able, incidentally, to evaluate our methods.

The more I thought about the MRC rejection of our project the more determined I became. Why, if we were successful, and we fully expected to be successful eventually, we would open up the whole world of human embryology. There would be new approaches in medicine. We would bring hope to thousands upon thousands of infertile women and there might well be all kinds of other benefits to human kind.

'What has the MRC done in the past few years to offer such hope?' I said to Ruth. 'They've spent hundreds of thousands of pounds on mouse, rat and rabbit embryos. Some of their single grants have been double, treble, the amount we could manage on. And apart from some highly specialized fields of research to what avail has all that money been spent?'

There was no point in being bitter. Though we were on the floor we had to pick ourselves up. Things were made more difficult for us because the decision of the Medical Research Council was leaked to the national press – I have never understood who leaked it nor the reasons why. We reported the situation to the Ethical Committee of the Oldham General Hospital – this consisted of a senior surgeon, a pathologist, a clergyman, a psychiatrist and a councillor. They maintained their support for us. Generously, they took their own independent decision. The Oldham Area Health Authority indeed did us proud, offering us when we requested it accommodation at Kershaw's Cottage Hospital in Royton. It was a small hospital two miles north of Oldham and was used, from time to time, by general practitioners who periodically admitted their patients there. We were allowed use of the operating area and three tiny rooms adjacent to it which, with the grant the Authority gave us, we transformed into a small laboratory, a culture room and an anaesthetic room. We installed working surfaces, sinks, ultraviolet lights for sterilization, gas services and other necessary additions. Also there were bedrooms for us and a bed-sitting room. We were in business again. We had our own clinic-cum-laboratory organized and planned specifically for our work. And we had the full cooperation of the matron, Mr Holmes and his staff.

Yet we needed more money to introduce sterile air, washable walls, clean surfaces, microscopes, balances, incubators, all the accoutrements needed for culturing our embryos. Patrick bought some of his equipment himself – operating tables and so on – but how we could have done with State funds! Now here's the ironic thing – the publicity that had irritated us so much suddenly worked in our favour: it attracted private supporters to our cause, generous individuals, mostly American. Thanks to them, we were donated enough cash to cover even such matters as car-hire providing we watched over general expenses carefully. In fact, it was doubly ironic. Here was I, a member of the Labour Party, supported in Royton by private enterprise and in Cambridge by the Ford Foundation.

When we resumed our work a routine soon became established. Patrick would start the treatment – injecting the hormones two or three days before Jean and I left Cambridge. It was the old drive north for us. We had to arrive there in time for the laparoscopy. Kershaw's led to more difficulties for Patrick and his staff. They had to quit their own operating theatre facilities at the Oldham General Hospital and bring all the extra equipment they needed to Kershaw's. Once the eggs had started on their indomitable ripening programme no hesitations were allowed. There was no turning back. Patrick had to be prepared to carry out the laparoscopy to obtain the eggs; Jean and I had to be at

Kershaw's on the dot to collect those same eggs prior to fertilization.

Alas, we discovered slowly that we were fertilizing fewer eggs than had been the case at Oldham. Cleavage too was less good. As a result Jean and I too often drove back to Cambridge silent and deflated, having achieved little or nothing though we had stayed several days up north. When we did obtain the embryos we had to flatten them on a glass slide again. That was a depressing job. But it was necessary to stain the chromosomes and, under the microscope, count the nuclei. We had to examine a sufficient number of embryos in order to exclude the chance of an abnormality.

'It's slow going,' I told Patrick, 'we'll be away lecturing at a meeting in Tokyo in October. It's a very important occasion for us.'

'At this rate,' Patrick said, 'we won't be replacing our first embryo until 1972.'

When the time came to replant the embryo into the mother's womb we would have to decide whether to inject it through the wall of the womb or to use the body's own channel – through the cervix and into the womb. The former method would require the patient to have a general anaesthetic for the abdomen would be opened or a laparoscope introduced. That was undesirable, especially as our patient would already have had, only a few days earlier, one general anaesthetic when laparoscopy was performed to obtain the eggs for fertilization. Also there was the potential damage the needle could cause in penetrating the thick wall of the womb. The second alternative therefore seemed preferable, safer, and less disturbing for the patient.

On the other hand I was aware of the recent results of those veterinarians and experimental scientists who had been successful in taking the fertilized embryo from the inside of one cow and transferring it into the womb of another. These transfers had more often failed when they had used the simpler natural route to the womb. Not many of the recipient cows became pregnant. What was true for farm animals might be true also for human beings.

'Maybe, but we don't want our patients to undergo abdominal surgery,' Patrick said. 'I can easily pass a fine catheter through the cervical canal then introduce the embryo back into the mother. She'd require no anaesthetic for that.'

So we decided that we would, when the time came, use the natural route. Meanwhile, in October, I received a series of insistent transatlantic telephone calls from Sargent Shriver, brother-in-law of John Kennedy. He pressed me to visit Washington. Round table discussions on ethics in medicine were to take place and one was to be devoted to fertilization *in vitro*. Shriver made it clear to me that this symposium was supported by the Kennedy Foundation in Washington and would be a most important event. All kinds of distinguished people would attend – senators, judges, doctors, scientists, writers.

'I'm sorry,' I said over the phone, 'but I've already accepted an invitation to attend another meeting in Tokyo.'

Another telephone call from my old friend Howard Jones, at Johns Hopkins in Baltimore, finally made me change my mind. 'If you could make a detour through Washington on your way to Tokyo it would be a great fillip to the work on fertilization in the USA,' that, from Howard, persuaded me.

Thus at the last possible moment I boarded a plane destined for Dulles Airport, Washington DC. Jet-lagged, I arrived just in time for a magnificent dinner at the Shrivers' on the night before the symposium opened. Among the guests were many renowned scientists as well as famous figures like Mother Teresa of Calcutta and Jean Vanier, founder of villages for the handicapped. James Watson was also present. Over dinner he was less than jocular.

The work Watson had carried out at Cambridge years earlier was beautiful. He had discovered the double helix structure of DNA, the molecule governing heredity, and for this he had won the Nobel Prize. He had written articles on our work and had become all heated up about cloning, fearing that we might go in that direction. Another guest I spotted who was opposed to our work was Leon Kass of the National Academy of Sciences. He had argued that our work was not therapeutic – women would still be infertile even if we successfully produced live children after reimplanting embryos in them. That argument surely was scarcely credible. So much medical treatment is directed towards replacing a deficiency rather than producing a cure. Consider, for instance, the life-saving therapy of insulin for diabetes. Or, for that matter, the value of false teeth and spectacles!

Next morning, desperately short of sleep, I joined the panel that was to take part in the discussion entitled, 'Fabricated babies: the ethics of the new technology in beginning life'. On the panel were James Watson, Leon Kass and Howard Jones. Also Paul Ramsey, a theologian from Princeton University, Anne McLaren, a British embryologist and David Daube, an academic lawyer from Harvard. The chairman invited me to speak first and I made a short opening statement to the very large audience which had assembled. Knowing some of the opinions of those on the panel I decided to sit back and wait to counter-attack.

Ramsey then rose to speak. He had to be seen and heard to be believed. I had to endure a denunciation of our work as if from some nineteenth-century pulpit. It was delivered with Gale 8 force, and written in similar vein a year later in the *Journal of the American Medical Association*. He doubted that our patients had their fully understanding consent. We ignored the sanctity of life. We carried out immoral experiments on the unborn. Our work was, he thundered, 'unethical medical experimentation on possible future human beings and therefore it is subject to absolute moral prohibition'. I was as much surprised as made wrathful by this impertinent scorching attack. He abused everything I stood for.

Kass then followed him and suggested that babies created by artificial fertilization may well be deformed in the process. 'It doesn't matter how many times the baby is tested while in the mother's womb,' he averred, 'they will never be certain the baby won't be born without defect.'

When James Watson was introduced it was evident the audience was listening now with an almost tangible expectancy. They had all heard of James Watson of the Double Helix.

'You can only go ahead with your work,' Watson addressed me, 'if you accept the necessity of infanticide. There are going to be a lot of mistakes.' He turned towards the audience and his voice became harsher. 'What are we going to do with the mistakes? We have to think about some things we refuse to think about.' These words were printed widely, in the *Guardian*, *Times* and *Daily Telegraph* in the UK on the following days.

Then Anne McLaren of Edinburgh University was invited to contribute to the discussion. She approved of our work generally, yet she said, 'I fear Dr Edwards will go too far, too fast. I am worried by the possibility that the desire to be first in the field will bias the judgement of those in a position to carry out egg transfer.' How could I reply to that? By saying flatly that her worries had no foundation in fact and that we were taking every care? 'However, babies produced in a test-tube,' she continued, 'will be routine procedure within twenty years.' Our patients admitted to Kershaw's would hardly find inspirational joy in that prognostication.

Howard Jones rose to defend our work, pouring scorn on the suggested moratorium on it and saying that the criticisms we had to experience were like 'the tribulations of Galileo'! Finally Daube insisted that the law should remain neutral – it should leave the decisions to scientists and doctors. That certainly was a new angle as far as I was concerned. So now all the panel had spoken. The Chairman invited me to reply.

I decided to deal with Ramsey first. I would let him have it. I was a Yorkshireman and I would be blunt as Yorkshiremen are reputed to be. He had uttered sentiments in his rhetorical way that would not have disgraced those directed against Charles Darwin one hundred years earlier. There was a hush as I rose to speak. I became aware of it. I heard the continuous soft sound of an air conditioner, and then I said sharply:

'I accuse Paul Ramsey of taking up an ethical stance that is about one hundred years out of date and one that is totally inapplicable to meet the difficult choices raised by modern scientific and technological advance.' I had hardly begun my second sentence – 'Dogma that has entered biology either from Communist or from Christian sources has done nothing but harm . . . .' – when I was interrupted by huge applause. The audience were on their feet clapping. I was amazed. Startled. I did not know how this loud spontaneous response affected Ramsey but as I glanced down at him at that moment and as the applause continued I felt sorry for him. His point of view had been shatteringly rejected by the audience. Indeed he made no further contribution to that symposium.

I then argued against Kass and Watson. I expressed my own opinion about the ethical aspects of our work. I related the numerous experiments on early mammalian embryos, and I mentioned our care and concern for our infertile patients and for their future babies. 'Our work will continue,' I said. 'This plea for our experiments to stop is an ultra-conservative one and unacceptable . . . . '

I missed the debates with reporters and newsmen in Washington; I had to fly to Tokyo immediately, even before the conference ended. In the plane I wondered about James Watson. He appeared to be concerned about any 'mistakes' we may make. His studies on DNA paved the way for genetic engineering. *There* is a subject fraught with potential dangers, and its ethical issues are now coming home to roost as genetic engineering is being applied to microorganisms. In the *Washington Post* of 14 May 1978, he wrote: 'I most certainly am a friend of DNA and want work with recombinant DNA to go as fast as possible . . . . all we know about infectious diseases makes it unlikely that the addition of a little foreign DNA will create any danger for those who work with recombinant DNA-bearing bacteria . . . . DNA is frequently carried from one species to another by viruses, and the global evolutionary impact of our experiment must be negligible compared to naturally occurring DNA transfers.' And all this despite the potential dangers which raise fears and objections in many environmentalists and geneticists like Pamela Lippe, who wrote later in the same paper that '. . . . unfortunately there is little, if any proof of Dr Watson's assertions of absolute safety'. Perhaps Watson now finds himself in a position not unlike mine in 1971. He too, has to face problems, to weigh every ounce of knowledge in the balance in order to reach a further conclusion.

Though certain of the justice of our work, it would be wrong to pretend that all the hostility that Patrick and I were from time to time subjected to – whether in London or Washington – left us entirely unaffected. The decision of the Medical Research Council not to support us had become common knowledge. Though that decision had been made by those with little awareness of our work, it sustained our critics. We had continued to report our progress in the *Lancet* and *Nature* and each successive paper sparked off a crescendo of debate. I have described but one symposium in Washington in some detail. I could have written about many others where I had to face equally difficult opposition.

On the other hand I would not wish the reader to imagine we were over-vulnerable. I had been a member of a small committee for some years now that had been formed to clarify ethical issues arising from advances in biology. Its Chairman was Walter Bodmer, Professor of Genetics at Oxford University. It included a theologian, Gordon Dunstan, John Maddox, who was the editor of *Nature*, and two politicians, Shirley Williams, a future Cabinet Minister, and David Owen, a future Foreign Secretary. Doctors and scientists like myself held numerous meetings and we called on many witnesses to discuss organ transplantation, the screening of foetuses for inherited disorders, artificial insemination and, of course, fertilization *in vitro*. Some of the independent-minded men and women of that committee, including Anne McLaren, had decided for themselves during our deliberation that fertilization *in vitro* was safe and ethical. No, I'm not trying to say that it was Patrick and Jean and I against the whole world!

Soon the aeroplane was taking me back to England. I did not know then how soon it would be before we would replace our first embryo into its mother nor how this would be attended by failure. I was looking forward only to returning to my wife and to seeing my children. Ruth would be interested to hear about the meetings, especially the one in Washington. At London's Heathrow, I collected my baggage which contained presents for the family and made for the customs barrier.

16
Bad Days in Oldham
Robert Edwards

On my return home in late October 1971 I did not have to tell Ruth about the assaulting speeches made in Washington. Reports of the meeting had been printed in the British national newspapers. Moreover the *Cambridge Evening News* had been busy, one of its reporters having telephoned scientists and others for a comment on James Watson's attack on our work. He had telephoned Jean Purdy but she had declined to comment. Max Perutz, another Nobel Prize winner in molecular biology and a fellow don in Cambridge, had responded, however. The newspaper was still hanging around the house and Ruth handed it to me.

I read: 'A warning that research into the production of "test-tube" babies may have "horrifying" consequences similar to the thalidomide catastrophe was given today by Nobel Prize winner and one of Cambridge's foremost scientists, Dr Max Perutz. Dr Perutz whose Nobel Prize was shared with another Cambridge don for work on blood and muscle haemoglobin, was commenting on criticism in America of the work of Cambridge scientist Dr Robert Edwards who is aiming to implant a fertilized ovum into the human uterus . . . . Dr Perutz said, ". . . . I agree entirely with Dr Watson that this is far too great a risk. Even if only a single abnormal baby is born and has to be kept alive as an invalid for the rest of its life, Dr Edwards would have a terrible guilt upon his shoulders. The idea that this might happen on a larger scale – a new thalidomide catastrophe – is horrifying . . . ." '

'People should know better than that,' I said, putting down the paper.

'All the same Bunny Austin sent a long letter to the paper,' Ruth told me, 'answering his criticisms point by point.' Some years later Perutz told me how surprised he was that a few words over the phone to a newspaper had led to such instant publicity. How could I reply to such a statement from a man in a high public position? And five years later when I was a councillor on the Cambridge City Council, I heard from a worried colleague that ironically genetic engineering was to be undertaken in Perutz's laboratory, funded by the Medical Research Council, and sited next to a major hospital. Sauce for the goose?

I never belittled the strength of feelings that some have had about our work on early human embryos. I respected the right of others to differ from my own standpoint. Nevertheless some remarks made on fertilization *in vitro* of human eggs appeared unworthy of serious consideration.

In November and December I journeyed to Oldham a number of times, and just before Christmas I felt we could go ahead and replant our first embryo into its mother. For we had examined enough fertilized ova and their nuclei had been excellent, the numbers of chromosomes in each cell as we had hoped. The blastocysts had been as lovely as ever. We knew that only one spermatozoon was penetrating the egg and that fertilization had been normal.

I decided that the best thing would be to replace the embryo into the mother when it had eight cells – usually two and a half days after fertilization.

'I want to get it back into the mother as soon as possible,' I told Patrick, 'as soon as the uterus will welcome the embryo.'

From now on our patients would not have to volunteer for laparoscopy only. Our work was becoming a clinical reality. How pleased the patients would be when Patrick explained to them that we would now be admitting them in the hope of establishing their own pregnancy. Of course they would have to understand the novelty of their treatment and how nobody could foretell their chances of pregnancy. Everything would be put to them – how, with their agreement, we would, if pregnancy took place, examine the foetus throughout the whole term of gestation – especially at sixteen weeks when we would carry out that chromosomal check-up. For we had to proceed cautiously.

Each patient had to have the best possible treatment and we could not proceed in the usual scientific way of establishing control groups, allowing others different treatment – different timing in the procedures for instance. We had to use one method, carefully modify it one degree at a time and so find out if any improvements were at all possible. The progress of each patient would have to be followed by endless assessments of her hormone levels, and any changes scrutinized closely to see if there were any signs of early pregnancy.

So with a sense of an important occasion Patrick passed the embryo in its drop of culture medium and in a cannula gently through the cervical canal of our first hoped-for mother. There was a few seconds' delay while the fluid dispersed and the embryo was carried into the recesses of the womb.

A quick check then under the microscope to make absolutely sure the embryo had left the cannula, and that was all. It had been performed cleanly, efficiently, simply, under sterile conditions and in a matter of a few minutes. By the middle of January 1972 we knew that our patient was not pregnant. It takes up to two weeks to elapse after replanting the embryo before one can be certain that the method has failed. But we would try again. We would, in the future, replace embryos in two, or even three, patients during a session at Kershaw's. Jean and I would then return to Cambridge and await events and reports from Patrick in Oldham.

Our initial replacements were unsuccessful. Some patients gave themselves and us hope because of a long interval before their next period, but not one of them became pregnant. The hormone tests we were doing confirmed our failures. Nor could we proceed as swiftly as we hoped. We were still not achieving fertilization as frequently as had been the case before we came to Kershaw's. And some embryos displayed poor cleavage.

'Why?' asked Patrick.

'I don't know,' I replied.

Then I saw Patrick's face. He was obviously in pain. 'Are you all right?' I asked him. Patrick had arthritic hips and they seemed to be getting worse. He had increased difficulty in standing for long periods and in walking.

At home too the conditions of our life were altering a little. Ruth wanted to undertake work of her own. With a family of five daughters she had not had time to use her considerable scientific skills, although she had been a great·help to me, supportive in every way and we had written joint papers to the *Scientific American* and other journals. Now, though, our youngest, the twins were eight years of age and going to school. Ruth felt she was able to apply for a Gulbenkian fellowship at Lucy

Cavendish College. Much to her surprise she obtained an award and so started part-time research in the Department of Investigative Medicine situated only some twenty yards down the road from my own laboratory.

In May I stood for election to the Cambridge City Council. I doubt if Patrick or Jean was pleased when they heard I had been successful and so had become a city councillor. They felt that local politics, my involvement with the affairs of the local community, might distract me from our singular goals in Oldham. It would not – but all the same I wished that I knew the reason for the relative infrequency of our achieving fertilization.

Even today I am unsure of why, during 1972, we were so much less successful than we had been earlier. Perhaps we had modified our culture fluids without realizing it, made some imperceptible change each time we journeyed to Kershaw's hospital – all the minimum alterations accumulating into a series of progressive small faults that drastically reduced our success rate. The move to Kershaw's itself may have worked against us. Fired with enthusiasm, and a desire for a fresh start, we had purchased new samples of chemicals, new drugs, new compounds, discarding the old ones that had stood us in good stead. Chemicals and drugs vary from sample to sample. It is a wise man who jealously conserves a preparation known to work.

I had not given up the idea of obtaining some State funds to support our work. A good opportunity came when a small group from our Committee chaired by Walter Bodmer went to see Dr David Owen, then Minister of Health in the Labour Government. The meeting had been arranged to discuss various implications in the advances in medicine. Such issues had been ventilated in our earlier meetings in London and then David Owen had been sympathetic.

'I'll have a crack at raising the whole business of State support for our work,' I told Jean one day as we drove back from Oldham after a depressingly unsuccessful session.

Most of the meeting was concerned with obtaining organs for transplantation from men and women who had been killed accidentally. Finally a moment did come that seemed propitious and I tackled the Minister about State support for fertilization *in vitro*. He responded bluntly, negatively: no help would be forthcoming. 'What a contrast,' I thought, 'to when he attended the meetings of our small Committee in London. Now he has the power but nothing will come from the Ministry.' I wondered what those United Nations Declarations on Human Rights meant, among them the right to establish a family. We would obviously have to rely on our existing resources to help our patients establish theirs.

These were, indeed, the bad days in Oldham. Nothing seemed to go right for us. We were still not as successful as we used to be in effecting fertilization; our attempts to establish pregnancy with blastocysts which we did manage to culture failed; and Patrick's arthritis became progressively worse. His limping gait became distinctive. We could hear him clumping, with a measured beat, down the long corridor of Kershaw's and we guessed that soon he would be needing a stick.

'If Patrick can't carry on,' Jean said one day to me, 'I suppose it will be curtains for us at Kershaw's?'

Patrick was due to retire in July 1978. I had hoped that we had at least till then to pursue our goals at Kershaw's.

For a moment I believe we both thought of Patrick. 'Have you noticed,' Jean said gently, 'when you talk to Patrick on the phone he always manages to put down the receiver before you do? He never really says goodbye on the phone.' I looked at Jean. She was not complaining; on the contrary, she was thinking of Patrick affectionately. 'Golly,' she added smiling, 'one of these days I shall manage to beat him to it.'

Despite everything, Kershaw's remained a happy place. It was not only the good nature and dedication of the staff. The women patients had so much in common with each other. They enjoyed each other's company. They understood and sympathized in a particularly poignant way with each other's common predicament. They came to Kershaw's with little hope. They witnessed the disappointments of those patients who preceded them in the treatment. True, some left Kershaw's with handkerchiefs clutched tightly in their hands but even then, with brimming eyes, they would stammer, 'We would not have missed the experience, doctor.' We would console them and promise to try again at a later date. Their disappointments did not leave us unaffected. Jean was particularly good with the patients. As an ex-nurse and as a woman she was clearly able to identify herself with them in a special way. She would sometimes point out small but important things that Patrick and I, as mere men, had overlooked.

We gradually realized why our endeavours were being unsuccessful. The fertility drugs we prescribed had the unexpected
effect of shortening the menstrual cycle, often by almost a week.
By the time we had collected the eggs, fertilized them, let them
grow to the blastocyst stage, the womb was preparing to shed its
lining – to menstruate. So it would not retain the embryo. On
the other hand, if we did not give our patients the fertility drugs
there would be only one egg per menstrual cycle to aspirate from
its follicle, one egg to fertilize *in vitro*. A too difficult task. This
was our dilemma. It was not clear what we should do.

Of course we could have taken an egg from, say, Mrs A who
had been given the fertility drugs, fertilized it with the sperm of
Mr B and then transferred the resultant blastocyst into the womb
of Mrs B who would not have received fertility drugs. Then
without a doubt Mrs B would become pregnant – only the baby
growing inside her would not have been her own, though her
husband would have been the father.

Patrick, seeing how much his patients longed to have babies,
toyed with this idea of embryo transfer. It would be a form of
artificial insemination. Mrs B, right from the beginning almost,
would nurture the growing foetus in her own womb and it
would grow and grow until nine months later she would give
birth to the son or daughter of her own husband. Surely such a
baby would be much loved by Mrs B? There were too many
snags though. We did not know enough about the psychological
relationships between parents, recipients, and children. There
could be legal as well as moral problems too. It was much too
complicated.

'We'd better not,' I said. 'I'm against it.'

'I suppose you're right,' said Patrick.

So we continued with the fertility drugs and patiently renewed
our old endeavours. But soon our continued setbacks discouraged
Jean and me from making too many journeys to the north. And
when, in addition, a serious illness in Jean's family meant that
she was not able to join me to travel to Kershaw's the work there
came to a halt. Jean's cooperation had become crucial. It was no
longer just Patrick and me. We had become a threesome.

There was a gap of nine months when we never visited
Kershaw's at all. Friends of ours – Mike Ashwood-Smith, for
instance, or such colleagues as David Whittingham who had
worked with me in Cambridge since the early 1970s – asked,

'What progress are you making, Bob?' and I had to say, 'None. No progress at all.' As likely as not I would change the subject, and steer the conversation towards politics. For, more and more, I had become engrossed by the political situation in Britain in the winter of 1973-4. All our lives had become affected by Ted Heath's confrontation with the miners. These were the cold, dark days of the three-day week.

I knew where my sympathies lay. With the miners! This was the class struggle, naked and simple. I was a Labour councillor and the Prime Minister's bungling of the conflict had made me wish I could be a Member of Parliament. Yes, I decided I would like to become a Labour MP. Ruth was not too sympathetic towards such ambitions. 'For five years,' she said drily, 'you've been away so often from home rushing up to Oldham. Now if you became an MP you'd have to rush away to London.'

Despite Ruth's legitimate complaints I continued to hope that I would become the Cambridge candidate for the Labour Party. There were fellow Labour councillors who gave me every encouragement. I made my bid in the late summer of 1974, just failing to unseat the sitting candidate. Perhaps it was this failure that redirected me once more to my primary quest and forced me to concentrate on human embryology. It was as if I had had a sabbatical from Oldham, from all those journeys north. Now I was ready to start again, refreshed, to try to solve the dilemmas at Kershaw's. Yes, something had to be done about the patients there. At least one improvement had occurred – the new roads northwards were straight and wide. Jean and I could now drive to Oldham in three hours without speeding. And so we did. I decided that since we had taken over the first part of the menstrual cycle of our patients by giving them fertility drugs it would be worthwhile continuing to support it later on with hormones – that is to say, after laparoscopy. With hormones our patients would have a better chance of retaining the implanted blastocyst. But which hormones to give?

I thought about this again as Jean and I went for one of our long walks through the lovely countryside and villages near Royton. We often walked across the moors or through Delph, Daisy Nook, Uppermill or Dingley Dell. 'In our situation,' I told Jean, 'every doctor would give the patients more HCG.'

For years we had used that hormone to ripen eggs; but it had another role in women. It sustains the earliest stages of pregnancy and helps the embryo through its formative period. If we gave this hormone to the patient after the replacement of an embryo perhaps it would stimulate the womb to become more receptive to the implanted blastocyst.

Patrick agreed. Soon we were trying out this new routine, continuing, of course, with our hormone analysis and double-testing to see whether pregnancy had occurred. Our progress again was slow: we had to wait for one group of patients to begin their menstruation before we commenced treatment with another. We needed to discover everything possible about the changes in the womb. A complete knowledge of these alterations would surely provide us with the key to our problems.

Alas, the HCG did not work – nothing was successful. True, the HCG lengthened the menstrual cycle a little but it set the other natural ovarian hormones awry – the oestrogen and pro-gesterone. We tried adding compounds similar to oestrogen and progesterone to the treatment. No use. Not one of our patients became pregnant.

In the courtyard of Kershaw's, between the blaze of tulips on each side of us, Patrick and I discussed what we should do.

'Perhaps we should increase the amounts of progesterone and oestrogen,' I suggested.

I noticed Patrick flinch. He was obviously in pain. I felt so sorry for him. Sometimes it seemed to me that my friend could hardly stand, never mind walk. It was a disaster for such an active surgeon. Yet he never complained.

'Yes, we'll increase the dosage,' Patrick agreed.

So we walked back very very slowly into Kershaw's. Patrick murmured, 'Hip-replacement therapy is my best bet. I hope to have the operation before the end of this year.'

During that late spring and early summer we prescribed more progesterone, more oestrogen, or related compounds, for our patients after we had replanted their embryos. We tried a dozen times. One after one we had to admit at least a temporary defeat, had to telephone an anxious waiting husband and say, 'Sorry – we've failed again.' T. S. Eliot has remarked on those who are undefeated only because they go on trying. It was only in that sense that we were now undefeated.

No wonder I looked forward to the summer break when, for a time, there would be no more concrete disappointments. I had planned to go away with Ruth and the family to a farmhouse called Bruntscar in the Yorkshire Dales where I had spent the summers of my childhood. For some years we had rented this house – and I was, now, frankly looking forward to being away from the stress and tears of Kershaw's.

In late June, Jean and I travelled to the north for our last session before the break. Eight patients had been admitted. Once more, with hardly any expectancy of success, we replaced the blastocysts into their wombs and later prescribed the progesterone and oestrogen hormones.

First it was failure with Number 1 patient. Then Number 2 and Number 3. Afterwards it was the turn of Numbers 4, 5 and 6 to look downcast. We felt cheerless ourselves as we replaced our last two embryos. Soon Jean and I were preparing to return to Cambridge. We bade farewell to the two remaining patients who were to receive their hormones in five or six days' time. Then we were outside in the car, and driving home to Cambridge. I peered at the curving road ahead. Soon I would be free of hospitals, of the University laboratory, of the ever-ringing telephone. I would be in Bruntscar, hay-making, building stone walls, walking in the hills.

Bruntscar came true. Summer day of 1975 followed summer day slowly, with the buzz of a fly on a window pane. I watched high clouds in the blue skies sail over adagio and I began to feel relaxed. Kershaw's was a million miles away. On another planet. Then, one afternoon I was coming back from helping a neighbouring farmer who was sheep-dipping when I saw Mr Mason, the husband of the postmistress, cycling away from our farmhouse. He did not see me. I watched him for a moment as his bicycle disappeared down the road through the pastures and meadows. I wondered why he had been to our house. Usually letters arrived during the morning and were delivered by the postman in his red van.

'Hullo,' I shouted as I opened the front door of the farmhouse.

'There's a telegram for you,' called Sarah.

I went into the living room. There was the yellow envelope on the mantelpiece next to the clock where Ruth had put it after Mr Mason gave it to her. Had something happened in Cambridge? I did not open it immediately. I sensed that there might be some message in it that would curtail my holiday. Ruth came in from the kitchen. I was still holding the envelope. 'Aren't you going to open it?' she asked. It was from Patrick. 'PREGNANCY TEST

POSITIVE STOP RING ME URGENTLY STOP PATRICK.'

I looked up. Both Ruth and Sarah were staring at me.

'Anything wrong?' asked Ruth.

'No,' I said. 'It's marvellous.' Then I heard my own voice become loud. 'It's really marvellous.'

I handed the telegram to Ruth.

17
The Wind of Change

Robert Edwards

Had I worn a hat I would have thrown it in the air. Almost four years of attempting to implant embryos into their mothers' wombs without success, and now this abrupt news of a positive pregnancy test.

On the phone to Patrick I said, 'Presumably it's the extra hormones that have done the trick.'

'Presumably,' replied Patrick and he chuckled.

I chuckled too. We were both delighted. The fertility drugs had allowed us to collect many eggs but they had changed the conditions inside the womb so that the blastocyst could not become embedded there and grow. The extra-powerful hormones we had injected into our patients had neutralized these deleterious effects and, hey presto, a pregnancy had occurred.

'And we can help sustain this pregnancy by continuing with the hormone injections,' I said.

'Yes,' Patrick said. 'We are continuing to do so.'

'I'll ring you in a day or two,' I said.

'Fine,' Patrick replied.

At Kershaw's they would take careful recordings of the hormones in our patient and I would want to know the results. I would be telephoning Patrick regularly during the rest of my holiday. I left the telephone booth that was situated outside the Hill Inn. The pub would be opening soon. Perhaps I would wait and drop in for a celebratory drink? I noticed a wind had sprung up, making the leaves in the trees shuffle and somewhere I could hear a door banging. On this occasion I did not delay for a beer. Instead I walked the mile and a half back to the farmhouse thinking about our breakthrough at Kershaw's, the wind in my face. It was surely the wind of change!

After each telephone call to Patrick I felt more and more

excited. All the indications and signs of pregnancy had become increasingly evident. There was no doubt about it: a foetus lay embedded in our patient's womb and hour by hour, day by day, week by week, it grew through the early stages of its life.

The Bruntscar vacation was over. Patrick took an ultrasonic scan of the foetus in the womb. All was well. After five weeks all was still well. After six, seven weeks all continued to be well. Then, suddenly, Patrick had his doubts.

'What do you mean?' I asked.

'I don't like the way the pregnancy is developing,' he said. 'The baby's position in the uterus.'

'What's wrong with its position?'

'It's rather high, and to one side.'

'Why do you think that is?'

'It could possibly be an ectopic pregnancy. I hope not – but I'm worried.'

By an ectopic pregnancy Patrick meant that the foetus might be growing, not in the womb itself, but in the Fallopian tube, or rather in the stump of the Fallopian tube adjoining the uterus. This stump had remained in our patient after the ravaging damage of infection and surgery done to it in earlier years. A foetus growing in a Fallopian tube means that it is situated in cramped conditions and is usually doomed to die. Worse, if it did prove to be an ectopic pregnancy this same foetus would threaten the life of the mother – for it could burst through the wall of the tube causing considerable bleeding into the abdominal cavity.

The patient had been admitted to Oldham General Hospital.

We went there together to see her. Patrick was cheerful enough with her. She was a charming, rather quiet lady, not given to displaying her emotions. But now she flashed us both a transparently unforced happy smile.

'Anything to report to me?' Patrick asked her.

'No – well, I do, sometimes, get a slight pain. But nothing much, doctor,' she admitted.

Afterwards, when we were alone, Patrick looked troubled. 'It's suspicious. There is vague swelling to one side of the womb,' he reported.

As the days passed Patrick became increasingly concerned. Another ultrasonic scan confirmed Patrick's suspicions: it seemed that somehow or other the tiny embryo had passed through the womb into the stump of that Fallopian tube and had attached itself there – to grow, to cause our patient occasional pains and soon, if left alone, to threaten her very life. Such an ectopic pregnancy is by no means rare. It is a problem familiar to all gynaecologists. Patrick could not allow the embryo to grow further and expand and rupture the tube. He would have to operate. A laparoscopy would prove absolutely whether his diagnosis was correct. He would be able to look into the abdomen at the Fallopian tube directly.

Patrick had to explain all this to our patient who, of course, like us, was utterly dismayed. Alas, at laparoscopy, our fears were confirmed – the embryo was in the stump of the Fallopian tube and it had to be removed there and then. This was the sudden end of our high hopes. And how sad it was for our patient. Her husband came to collect her. From the courtyard inside the hospital I saw the couple leaving together. They stopped and turned towards Patrick. 'Can we try again, doctor?' the husband asked. He nodded. Then we watched their car, after the doors had slammed, move forward and gather speed and quit the hospital.

It was depressing. And yet, on reflection, we had made a real advance. We knew now that the blastocysts we had grown in our culture fluids could become implanted and grow through the delicate early stages of life. It confirmed for us that replacing the embryo into the womb through the natural route of the cervical canal did not, in some way, jeopardize it. Frettings and worryings of this kind, all kinds of other similar small but real forebodings that had from time to time assailed Patrick and me were now dissolved. We had corrected the hormone problems resulting from the fertility drugs by virtually taking over the menstrual cycle after replanting the embryo. We would do the same with other patients. When we mulled over all this we experienced a great fillip to our spirits.

Yet one tiny but persistent question worried me: *Supposing the Fallopian tube was receptive to the embryo in a way that the womb itself wasn't? Was it just luck that the embryo had reached the Fallopian tube stump rather than staying in the womb which might have rejected it?*

These were questions we would be able to answer eventually. But now it was time to write up all our data on the ectopic pregnancy and send it to the *Lancet*. Ectopic or not, it was the first human pregnancy begun outside the mother. It would be a page in the textbook of medical history. It was important to announce our progress in the medical press and I carefully parcelled up our manuscript and despatched it to the editor.

A few days later it arrived back on my desk. The editor could see nothing new in the case history! I could not help recalling the similar rejection letter I had received from the *Lancet* years earlier when I had sent them my paper on ripening eggs. Once again I telephoned the editor, pointing out the novel nature of our report and the excitement it would surely arouse.

'You'll have to shorten it,' he said.

I had heard that remark before somewhere. 'Certainly,' I said.

So the paper on our first human pregnancy was ultimately published in this most prestigious of medical journals. At once, many realized that we were near a turning-point in our long series of investigations.

And yet the sceptics remained. Indeed, we had given them cause for some suspicion. For in our paper we had reported every detail – including how, when Patrick had performed the early laparoscopy to collect the ripening eggs, he had noted there had been six available for fertilization *in vitro*. But he had only managed to pluck out five – the other remaining egg had escaped Patrick's attention and had presumably been lost in the peritoneal cavity.

Now our critics, among them my friend Howard Jones in North Carolina, suggested the ectopic pregnancy was the result of this one misplaced egg that had somehow entered the Fallopian tube and then had been fertilized naturally when the husband and wife had had sexual intercourse

We knew they were wrong because the stump of the Fallopian tube was totally blocked and distorted, as Patrick had noted at that same early laparoscopy and was later able to confirm when he removed it along with the foetus. Besides, our patient had remained in hospital for the whole period of her treatment from before laparoscopy until several days afterwards. It would have been very difficult, given the circumstances, for her to have had intercourse during this time.

The best way to convince our critics was for us to gain further pregnancies. We did not have to wait long. Hormone changes in the urine of another patient into whom we had replanted her embryo told us of a second success.

'It can't be an ectopic pregnancy this time,' Patrick said

buoyantly. 'This patient has no remnants of Fallopian tubes whatsoever.'

Alas, again the patient had to suffer bitter disappointment. After a few weeks the hormones began to falter and decline. Even before Patrick could examine her by an ultrasonic scan the baby had gone. Whatever else, we were now certain of the value of the hormones in sustaining the readiness of the womb for the embedding of the blastocyst and its growth.

Encouraged by our successes, such as they were, I determined to discover why we did not obtain the high rates of fertilization and cleavage which we had done before the move to Kershaw's. Just before Christmas in 1975 I drove to Royton and spent four successive days and nights testing all our culture fluids, all the drugs, all the containers, everything else we used. Finally I discovered what was not quite right – one constituent, liquid paraffin, which we had used to suppress evaporation, had become toxic. That was at least one reason for our diminished rate of fertilization.

We obtained five embryos from our next patient. We re-implanted two of them, trying for twins – unsuccessfully as it turned out. 'Don't squash the others,' said Jean. 'We've flattened 101 and I doubt these will tell us anything new.' The other three we allowed to stay in our culture fluids. It was a stimulating piece of embryology. We wanted to see if they would pass beyond the blastocyst stage. One of them did. It escaped from its membrane, expanding just as it would have done had it been in a receptive womb. We watched it day by day with wonder. Monday, Tuesday, Wednesday, Thursday . . . . it grew for nine days. From the moment of fertilization nine days of growth!

The embryo was still a speck, only just visible in our culture dish, but for me it represented the crucial stages of human embryology, the actual moments when the foundations are being laid for the formation of the body's organs. Cells and tissues grew and moved, assuming new forms in readiness for the moment when the embryo would begin to take a recognizable shape. Normally, of course, the embryo would be developing in this way inside its mother's womb, but I was privileged to watch it in our culture dish with all its promise of further growth.

I have always wanted to understand more of our early growth. I have always wondered if these cells, as they begin their transformation into the organs and tissues of the human body, would offer us scope in medicine to understand and correct deficiencies and disorders in children and adults. And there, in that single expanding embryo in the culture dish, lay the promise of achieving these ambitions. As I prepared the embryo for analysis, I feared that it might die and take with it all the evidence of its nine days of growth. Little did I know that I would never see another such embryo from that day to this.

Patrick was not with us during this period. He was in Wrightington Hospital near Wigan undergoing hip surgery. Jean and I went to visit him. The operation was a fantastic success. After intensive care for one day they soon made him stand. A few days later he was walking. It was unbelievable how gradually the full use of his legs came back. Before the spring of 1976 he was entirely and remarkably his old self.

Meanwhile Patrick's affable senior registrar, Gordon Faulkner, carried out the laparoscopies. We stepped up our work now that we felt so close to real success. But over the next few months,

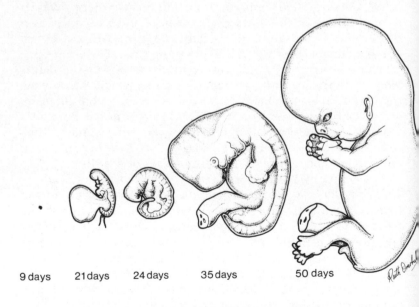

9 days   21 days   24 days   35 days   50 days

'It grew for nine days . . . . The embryo was still a speck, only just visible in our culture dish.' After that, the organs form – the cells gradually become capable of development into heart, lungs, brain, eye.

despite all our intensified efforts, only one of our patients became pregnant and then, alas, only briefly. It was a trying and frustrating time for our patients, who realized now how close we were to helping them. What a long slow haul they had to endure – the initial wait in hospital, the injections of hormones to stimulate the ripening of their eggs, then the laparoscopy, followed by more and different hormones that would prepare the womb to be receptive. And after all that, and after the tests to see if they were pregnant, the going home to a house generally without children's voices in it, going back from where they had set out with hope and returned in disappointment and with the taste of nothing on the tongue.

We had to do something especially now that Patrick was back and seemingly full of energy. We had identified the problem but had not solved it. The hormone supplements we had prescribed to sustain pregnancy had evidently done as much as they were going to do.

'And we can't give any higher doses to our patients,' asserted Patrick justly.

New and drastic departures from our routine were obviously needed. We had probably been lucky with the ectopic pregnancy. And we had managed to approximate the right conditions in two other patients. But this was not enough.

18

Back to Nature

Robert Edwards

'We would certainly increase the chances of pregnancy if we could get nearer to the natural events in the menstrual cycle,' I said to Jean. 'Still, if we abandon the fertility drugs and the HCG our problems will be formidable.'

We had left the lab and gone downstairs to the Common Room where we could sip some tea and relax and greet some of our colleagues of the Cambridge Physiological Laboratory. But as was so often the case I found myself discussing intensely with Jean ideas of what we should do at Kershaw's.

'If only we could manage it without all the drugs,' she said, 'wouldn't it be fantastic!'

Jean felt uneasy sometimes about the powerful hormones we had to give our patients in order to control their menstrual cycle. But we needed the fertility drugs to make the ovary super-ovulate. On the other hand, when on occasions these drugs had virtually failed, the ovary responding weakly, and there had been only one egg for the taking, Patrick, with all his skill, had managed it. The culture fluids too were once again richly working so that our rates of fertilization had become high. Yes, I felt confident that Jean and I could fertilize a single egg if Patrick could deliver it – and he surely would if only he knew when exactly to undertake the laparoscopy. If he went in too soon the egg would not have ripened sufficiently to yield us a good embryo; if too late that same egg would have burst out of the ovarian follicle to be irrevocably lost in the abdominal cavity.

'We would be on a tightrope,' I said.

Jean raised the cup to her mouth, nodding as she looked at me. There was one possible approach. I had a shrewd idea that maybe there was some signpost that could help us determine the exact time to catch the lone egg. For at a definite point in the menstrual cycle, usually about day 13, women suddenly discharge from a gland near the brain a certain hormone – the luteinizing hormone (LH) which brings about the ripening of the egg. So much LH is released into the bloodstream that an hour or so later LH spills over into the urine. This sudden discharge is aptly called the surge of LH. It really is a surge – the hormone doubles its levels of concentration in the bloodstream within so brief a period of time. If I could measure the LH in the urine, say, I would have a pointer when to suggest the laparoscopy.

'Yet even if we solved all that,' I continued, 'we'd be no longer controlling the menstrual cycle, merely observing it – and we would be tied mercilessly to the patient's menstrual and ovulation cycle. Laparoscopies at dawn – just imagine it!' I recalled those long ago days in Edinburgh when day and night I had been at the beck and call of the mice.

'What alternative is there?' Jean asked.

The Common Room had emptied. Even the ladies who served us tea or coffee had quit their bar. I glanced at the brightly coloured chairs waiting in their postures of expectancy. In this same Common Room I had frequently chatted to my ex-colleague David Whittingham. He had left us to continue his research at University College in Central London. Now I recalled how he had managed to freeze mouse blastocysts to incredibly low temperatures without harming them. Frozen at −196 degrees Centigrade and even at much lower temperatures they had been stored for months, then thawed out one by one, to be replaced into a host female who later gave birth to normal mice.

'There is an alternative,' I said to Jean. 'We could try freezing human embryos. We'd give the fertility drugs as usual to patients, collect the ripening eggs, fertilize them, then when the eggs have divided into sixteen or thirty-two cells we'd freeze them and keep them in store until the effects of the fertility drugs on our patients had long faded away and their menstrual cycles were back to normal. Then we could thaw the embryos out and replace them in their mother.'

Since the mother's menstrual cycle would now be normal her womb would be receptive and capable of sustaining the growth of the foetus. The idea suddenly excited me. Why, if that strategy worked, we could provide the mother with a whole family, spaced in the way she wished, just thawing out each embryo when desired.

For years I had been closely aware of freezing schemes to
preserve life. Nor was it a modern science-fiction fantasy. As long
ago as 1776 the great Dr John Hunter had admitted in a lecture
that he had taken two living carp and frozen them in a vessel
containing river water. When he thawed them out he saw
unhappily that the fish were dead. 'Till this time,' he confessed,
'I had imagined that it might be possible to prolong life to any
period by freezing a person in the frigid zone as I thought all
action and waste would cease until the body was thawed. I
thought that if a man would give up the last years of his life to
this kind of alternative oblivion and action, it might be prolonged
to a thousand years; and by getting himself thawed every
hundred years he might learn what had happened during his
frozen condition. Like other schemes, I thought I should make
my fortune by it, but this experiment undeceived me.'

Hunter's fantasy nowadays may seem a forlorn and absurd
one; but altogether less ambitious and more probable goals have
been reached in recent years. For instance, Audrey Smith, who
had been my colleague at the Mill Hill National Institute for
Medical Research, had successfully frozen spermatozoa in 1956
– and since then similar techniques have been used in cattle
breeding. Now it is not uncommon for frozen spermatozoa to be
thawed out and used to impregnate cows. Frozen spermatozoa are
also used in human donor inseminations in many centres.

At Kershaw's we were left with 'spare' embryos – those which
we would not be attempting to replace in the womb. Perhaps we
could try freezing them? I would discuss it, of course, with
Patrick. And with David Whittingham too.

I stood up. Jean had put her cup down. 'At one blow freezing
our embryos might solve all our problems,' I said. We left the
Common Room determined on a new course of action.

Initially we sent the 'spare' embryos to London for David
Whittingham to freeze. They went by express on the Inter-City
train of British Rail from Manchester. I have often wondered
what the guards on those expresses would have said if they had
known what was in the parcels that we solemnly handed to them
at Manchester railway station! David managed to freeze one or
two of them and even to thaw them out without a great deal of
damage, but it became obvious that sending the embryos to
London was not the right answer. There was too much vibration
– a cork could come off the container for instance – and we had

no control over temperatures. I told Patrick that we would have to freeze the embryos there and then at Kershaw's. Obviously it would be altogether more desirable if we could transfer the embryos straight from our culture fluid into the freezing mixture.

'Machines are available especially designed for freezing such things as embryos,' I said. 'We could hire one.'

Before we hired the remarkable freezing machine our colleagues in Cambridge gave Jean and me lessons in the technique. I became fond of the machine! It was a beautifully designed piece of apparatus assembled on a trolley, capable of freezing tissues either swiftly or gradually over a period of hours – as required – to incredibly low temperatures.

Now we had it sitting there like a god in a small room in Kershaw's. It huffed endlessly, pumping a bitterly cold gas into its freezing chamber, one puff at a time, blinking its green lights each time it exhaled. For a period of weeks we placed all the spare embryos inside it and set it going. Opening a door at night, peering into the dark room, the night nurses must have taken a step backwards when confronted by this hissing, winking, green light contraption that pumped out clouds of gas. Not to mention the shock it gave to the morning cleaners!

Alas, despite all its ingenuity, and despite all our efforts we had to abandon this new approach when we discovered that not one of the thawed embryos appeared capable of further growth.

'Well, no one can say we're not trying,' said Jean. 'It was a good idea.'

'It might be the basis of a good idea in the future,' I said, 'but now it's back to the old routine of the fertility drugs.'

We were to use the fertility drugs for only one more series of patients. Patrick and I had had another notion. Some British doctors had reported that a new drug, Bromocryptine, a valuable compound now used to stop lactation in women who do not wish to suckle their babies, elongated the menstrual cycle in those women who menstruated too soon. When premature menstruation occurred embryos did not have enough time to become implanted in the womb, and so such women would benefit if prescribed this 'wonder' drug.

'It sounds just what we need,' Patrick said.

We told the patients in Kershaw's, some of whom had been admitted there before and had experienced our failures, that we were going to try out Bromocryptine. So, for the last time, we

went through our old familiar routine of injecting the patients
with fertility drugs, then HCG, followed by a laparoscopy thirty-
two hours later. After the eggs had been fertilized and had
developed to blastocysts and had been replaced in the womb, we
gave our patients the new wonder drug. For nine months we
persisted with this approach, but to our dismay the Bromocryptine hardly changed the length of their menstrual cycles at all.
Certainly there was not a single pregnancy to reward us for all
our efforts. So it was goodbye, Bromocryptine.

It was summer 1977 and as far as I was concerned it was
goodbye to the fertility drugs too. So at last we abandoned them
as we had abandoned the idea of the frozen embryos. There was
no alternative but to collect the single egg ripening naturally
within the mother. It sounded all so simple – and yet in practice
would be so difficult. Over the years, driving back to Cambridge
with Jean, I had said after this or that failure, 'That is it. That is
definitely it.' And felt depressed enough to mean it. Later I would
have another idea and then would determinedly remark, 'If this
doesn't work this will be the last time, this will definitely be our
last trip north.'

Now it seemed we were as far from our goal as ever. Yet we
had travelled too far, however zig-zag our course, to give up. First
of all I would have to discover a method of measuring the
patient's surge of LH – the hormone that stimulated the ripening
process. I began to make enquiries. One of my friends, a London
gynaecologist whom I had met over the years at those meetings
about ethical problems – she was particularly involved with
artificial insemination – recommended me to try a Japanese
product.

'It's called Hi-Gonavis,' she said. 'A curious name.'

During the summer holidays, when I was walking once more
over the hills of the Yorkshire Dales, sometimes I would recall
my childhood days. Certain places, a tilt of a field, a sky pattern,
a farm building or a wall, evoked in me moods of nostalgia. Other
times, though, I thought about Hi-Gonavis and how it might
help us to determine the LH surge when we tested the urine. In
the Yorkshire Dales it was back to nature. In the autumn, at
Kershaw's, it was back to nature in another sense.

Hi-Gonavis, a piece of pure Japanese ingenuity, affected the
way cell particles settled in a urine solution. If a sample of urine
was LH-free, particles would fall through it swiftly; but if large

amounts of LH were present then the particles settled very slowly. It was all so simple and I could get a result in two hours. By testing the urine of a patient at three-hourly intervals we would be able to learn precisely when the LH surge began.

'We'll have to ask our patients to collect all their urine!' said Jean.

'Yes,' I said. 'And measure it. There's going to be plenty of tea drunk at Kershaw's!'

The Hi-Gonavis test would signal to us when the egg had begun to ripen in the ovary. I also reckoned that by analysing the urine for another hormone, oestrogen, we would be given a longer-term warning. Oestrogen concentrations rise in the urine until day 13 of the menstrual cycle. This oestrogen test, as it were, would give us an amber light; the Hi-Gonavis test for LH, a red one.

From my past experience of ripening eggs I estimated that the best time for laparoscopy would be twenty-four to thirty hours after the surge commenced. Given that red light we could then alert Patrick and his team in good time. We were confident of Patrick's ability to collect the single ripening egg and in our ability to fertilize it.

We explained our new approach to the first three patients we brought into Kershaw's. They drank the tea, we collected the urine. When we observed the LH surge of our first patient we knew that the next day, in the operating theatre, our judgement would be on trial. At last we judged that our first patient was ready for laparoscopy. Patrick and his team came over from Oldham General Hospital. Soon she was unconscious and the laparoscopy began, Patrick making his short incision near the lower edge of the navel. Then the laparoscope was introduced.

Would there be one large follicle in the ovary with an egg ripening inside it, approaching its moment of ovulation as we had estimated? We waited breathlessly for Patrick's pronouncement.

Yes, yes, there it was.

Would Patrick bring it out safely, this one and only egg? He gently inserted the aspirating needle into the ripening follicle and withdrew its contents. Since there was only one follicle to be aspirated, the laparoscopy was all over in a matter of minutes and I was able to examine the follicle's contents immediately under a microscope. As I bent to look down I heard Jean murmur,

'Well?'

'Got it,' I said delightedly. 'A beauty.'

There it was visible, illuminated, the one lovely ripening egg sitting contentedly in its nurse cells. Neither Patrick, Jean nor I said much. Of course we were thrilled that our estimates had been accurate so far and that Patrick had collected the one egg. But there were miles to go yet before we could truly feel triumphant. I transferred the egg into our culture fluid and added spermatozoa. We would have to wait eighteen hours to see whether that egg would be fertilized.

We knew that we were in business when it began its beautiful cleavage divisions – two cells, then four cells. We would wait for it to become eight-celled before replacing it in the mother. Meanwhile our second patient, a Mrs Lesley Brown, according to our Hi-Gonavis tests was ready for laparoscopy.

19

A Patient Called Lesley Brown

Patrick Steptoe

In the autumn of 1976 a letter arrived from Dr Ruth Hinton, who was the medical officer of the Bristol Central Health Clinic. She asked me if I would see a Mrs Lesley Brown and her husband. It seemed that this couple had wanted children for almost a decade but that Mrs Brown had blocked Fallopian tubes. In 1970, because of these Fallopian tube occlusions, Lesley Brown had been operated on at Bristol Royal Infirmary. 'The outer quarter of each diseased tube,' Dr Hinton wrote me, 'had been excised and cuff-like openings fashioned to maintain patency on both sides.'

The beautifully coordinated, though complicated, business of natural conception may be tragically prevented if the tubes are occluded as a result of an old infection. Surgery may reopen these Fallopian tubes but cannot restore the damage done to their muscles, or to the linings, or to the fine, hair-like processes of those linings, called cilia, which, under normal circumstances, can row an egg along the cavity of the tube towards the womb.

In short, restoring the patency of the Fallopian tubes does not, in itself, guarantee future conception. Even if, subsequently, conception does take place, the fertilized embryo, instead of progressing to the womb, occasionally may be retained in the reconstructed tube to grow there and become a dangerous ectopic pregnancy. Should the damage to the Fallopian tubes be truly severe plastic surgery on them is doomed to fail in more than 80 per cent of cases. Such unlucky patients, despite bold surgery in the course of a stressful operation, are thereafter compelled to accept their sterility.

Sadly Mrs Lesley Brown appeared to be one of the unlucky 80 per cent. Special X rays taken after the operation revealed the tubes to be shortened, swollen, distorted, and still completely blocked. The operation, performed at Bristol Royal Infirmary six years previously, had failed.

I noted from Dr Hinton's letter that Mrs Brown was now twenty-nine years of age. Importantly, her husband, John had been found to be fertile – indeed he already had a fourteen-year-old daughter by a previous marriage. Could Bob Edwards and I help her? If not, it was evident that Mrs Brown would be childless forever.

That autumn of 1976 I felt confident about things. The operation on my hips had been a wonderful success and we were making progress at Kershaw's. I had watched with fascination Bob growing the embryos. They were so beautifully well-formed that one day we were bound to be successful. That ectopic pregnancy of a year earlier had surely been but a singular unlucky incident. I felt a new approach with the fertility drugs would win through again. I wanted most of all to be able to help those patients of mine who had been given up as hopeless by other doctors. And was not Lesley Brown one such? I wrote to Bristol offering Lesley Brown an appointment to see me.

On one of those sunny, hazy, November afternoons I first met the Browns. Mr Brown proved to be a broad-shouldered, stocky man. I had the immediate impression of someone physically strong.

He spoke in a soft, West Country brogue that reminded me of the accents of my childhood companions in Oxfordshire. Now he told me how deep was their disappointment at the failure of past treatment, and how traumatic this failure had been for Lesley. As a result of it, and her continuing inability to become pregnant, she had become severely depressed.

'She'd be good at having a baby too,' John Brown added.

,He looked towards her with evident deep devotion. Lesley Brown had brown hair and matching shy brown eyes. At first, she seemed hesitant in answering my questions and I realized that her slowness of speech was governed by a carefulness not to mislead. I learnt that Lesley's depression had led to friction with John. She felt she was letting John down by not having a baby. Their marriage had nearly broken apart. She had even tried to persuade her husband to divorce her so that he might marry someone else who could give him a child. John would have none of that. Together, finally, they had sat down to write another pleading letter to Dr Hinton.

'I would be a good mother,' Mrs Brown said softly.

It was quiet in my consulting room before John Brown said feelingly, 'You see, doctor, she always wanted a child.'

I discussed Lesley's clinical condition with her before examining her in detail. I would need to do a laparoscopy, to scrutinize the ovaries and the pelvis directly to see the residual effects of Lesley's previous disease and of the operations she had experienced. After the clinical examination I explained this to her.

'It'll mean a brief stay in hospital,' I continued, 'and a short anaesthetic.'

I turned to John. I explained how we would need to make a special examination of his seminal fluid – this to be produced carefully and cleanly by masturbation, after a few days of sexual abstinence. I then outlined to the Browns, as I had to so many couples in the past, how, if all turned out well, at a later date I hoped to collect an egg and fertilize it *in vitro*. I explained all the concepts as simply as possible so that they fully understood.

'Yes,' I continued, 'if we do fertilize one of your eggs with John's spermatozoa and the resulting embryo grows normally and healthily during the next few days, we would then attempt to replace it into the body of the womb.'

'Would that require another anaesthetic?' John asked.

'No,' I said, 'but the position may be a little uncomfortable.'

I explained to them why we believed that if we were successful the abnormality rate among the offspring conceived by this means would be no greater than that following natural conception. I told them how, if pregnancy occurred, we could in any case find out about any serious abnormality – and if we did discover such an abnormality this would be dealt with by induced abortion.

'Such an event, however, is unlikely,' I told them.

During this initial consultation I was able to assess Lesley and John. He was devoted to her welfare and would not brook high risks to her. She was quietly determined, strong in resolve, unlikely to panic, and would suffer whatever was necessary with stoicism. They were an ideal couple for our attempted treatment – which I told them was only available under the National Health Service though there would be some delay in starting it.

'Our facilities are limited,' I explained. 'But within that constriction I hope to send for Lesley in a few months' time.'

In the event Lesley Brown was admitted to a hospital bed in

February 1977.

On 26 February, a laparoscopy was performed under general anaesthesia. The immediate view of the pelvis was startling. A bright yellow apron of fat – the omentum – obscured my field of vision because it adhered to the internal part of her abdominal scar. To either side of the apron, however, there were free spaces. By the cunning use of an angled lens through these gaps I was able to view the pelvic organs.

A large distorted pink mass obscured the left ovary and was stuck to it. This pink mass had formed from the left tube. Moreover a veil of adhesions covered the ovary also, fixing it to the back of the womb. As for the right side, I could see a short occluded stump of a tube. And this was fixed to the side wall of the pelvis in such a way that it could not be examined nor mobilized completely.

'An open operation will be needed,' I thought, 'to clear away the adhesions, to remove the remains of the diseased tubes, to free the ovaries.'

Such a surgical intervention could not be done right away. It would have to be timed carefully so that healing could take place undisturbed by menstruation. Poor Lesley Brown – she would have to wait before definitive treatment could be undertaken. I explained all this to her later. She nodded. She was stoical as I knew she would be. But the day after the laparoscopy she set out for Bristol against my advice because John had to return to work. I had wanted her to stay one more day in hospital to recover fully. In the event the tiny half-inch incision I had made began to bleed. It was hardly serious but a little blood can spread a long way. Certainly it upset and alarmed John on their long trek back to Bristol. The little wound soon healed quickly, after it had been cleaned up, and despite that mishap Lesley was determined to continue her treatment.

On 7 August Lesley again travelled to Oldham. The next day I opened her old scar, separated the yellow omental fatty apron from the internal scar, divided the numerous adhesions. At last, the ovaries with their diseased tubes were clearly revealed. I removed the blocked sepulchres of tubes completely and freed the ovaries. Towards the end of the operation a special solution was placed in the pelvis which would discourage any more formation of adhesions.

Lesley made a good recovery from this operation. She was

given antibiotics and steroids – the latter to further discourage adhesion formation – and eight days later she was ready to return to Bristol. All was well. Soon Lesley would be ready for an attempt at *in vitro* fertilization. Her menstrual cycle continued undisturbed and it was confirmed that John's semen was potentially fertile. Numerous healthy, mobile spermatozoa were present in a bacteria-free fluid.

It was about this time that Bob suggested we should abandon the fertility drugs we had used to obtain superovulation. He had already decided that we would have to give up the idea of storing embryos by freezing them and using them at a more favourable time when the patient's menstrual cycle had returned to normal.

'We'll just have to try recovering the ovum in its natural cycle at the right moment of its ripening,' Bob said.

We began to discuss the LH surge and the possibility of timing the laparoscopy. Would we be able to time it just before the follicle ruptured, and released the mature egg into the abdomen where it would be lost irrevocably? Even if Bob could solve this timing problem it would mean that I and all my team would be tied to the patients' menstrual and ovulation cycles.

'It could be day or night,' I said.

'Yes,' said Bob.

I nodded. I thought of Lesley Brown and other patients of mine. For the last five years particularly I had had to console them repeatedly. True, I had been frank with them all. They all knew that our approach was novel and unpredictable. But of course it did not help them when our method failed. We had to be successful. For their sake. There was no turning back now. One worry for me was that I had less than a year now before retiring.

'I retire next June,' I reminded Bob.

'I know.'

'But I think I could ask for a special extension of our use of Kershaw's,' I added, 'so that we can treat our last group of patients properly.'

20

The Minuscule Dot of Life

Patrick Steptoe

I parked the car outside Kershaw's. Then walked carefully, because of the slippery damp leaves on the pathway, into the little hospital where Bob and Jean were waiting for me. Bob had phoned me earlier, urging me to come over and see this new method of measuring the LH surge. 'This Hi-Gonavis is a beautifully packed kit. Typical Japanese ingenuity,' he had said. I was confronted with a series of little tubes full of red blood cells. They were scattered everywhere from the mantelpiece to the window sills.

Bob and Jean felt confident that they would now be able to tell me exactly when a laparoscopy would be worthwhile – their judgement based on the results of these little tubes. Weeks before they had squabbled about the best way of doing things. Now they had made up their minds and I was faced with their united view. The procedure could be awkward. It would no longer be possible to carry out operations when it suited me or my team. But Bob and Jean knew that Muriel Harris, my theatre supervisor, along with my anaesthetists and my nurses, would stand by me in any demand that I should make upon them. They were right. I was lucky to enjoy such generous loyalty.

One of the patients waiting for a laparoscopy at Kershaw's that autumn day was Lesley Brown. They had been testing samples of her urine as well as those of other patients with the Hi-Gonavis kits, and on 10 November 1977 at 11 a.m., twenty-six hours after the onset of her LH surge had been identified on the fifteenth day of her cycle, she was ready for laparoscopy. At the same time, John Brown produced a fresh semen specimen.

Clean sterile air was pumped into the laboratory and the preparation of a warm stage on the microscope completed. John's semen was examined and by spinning it in a centrifuge the spermatozoa separated from their plasma. The latter was removed and a carefully prepared culture medium put in its place. The concentration of spermatozoa was so adjusted that one millilitre of the mixture contained one million sperms. Droplets of the prepared semen were now placed under liquid paraffin in a Petri dish and then put in an incubator kept at normal body temperature. The vessel holding the Petri dish was capable of being filled with a special gas mixture which could maintain the balance between alkalinity and acidity – otherwise the sperm cells would be damaged. So John's spermatozoa were ready. Now we needed to recover the one ovum of Lesley's that was presumably ripening and ready to be collected.

Lesley had been anaesthetized by Dr Finlay Campbell. My assistant, Dr John Webster, had completed his preparations for the laparoscopy and now we were ready to begin. Lesley had been draped and a special needle was passed into the abdomen at the lower border of her navel so that a gas mixture, the same as that used for fertilization and cleavage, could be passed into the abdomen while the operating table was tilted head downwards about 20 degrees. The gas in the pelvis allowed a free safe space for larger instruments to be introduced while the intestines fell back out of the way.

When I introduced the laparoscope I could see that there had been some recurrence of adhesions around the ovaries despite the operative treatment given earlier to Lesley. Another instrument was introduced from the side of the abdomen and the womb and ovaries were mobilized by holding the supporting ligaments and by manipulating them. My heart sank. The right ovary contained three small follicles only. No pre-ovulatory follicle was there. Had Bob and Jean's estimations, with the help of the Hi-Gonavis kit, been wrong? Bob was no more than eight feet away from me on the other side of the door which separated the operating theatre from the culture laboratory. We had recently established an intercommunication system and I was tempted to say out loud my disappointment. But first I would view the left ovary which I was finding more difficult to mobilize. I had to remove carefully a small omental adhesion. And then – ah there it was, I could see it! – a ripe, pinkish-blue follicle. Yes, on the under surface of that left ovary a good ripe follicle about three centimetres in diameter.

'Bob, one good follicle in the left ovary,' I said, pleased, over the intercom. 'But not easy to approach. Adhesions.'

'I'm ready,' Bob replied.

To the left of the midline I introduced a sharp cannula some 2.2 millimetres in diameter. I then injected through it some anti-clot saline solution which would clean away any minute traces of fat and blood that might have entered it. Through the cleaned cannula I introduced a special long needle, 1.3 millimetres in diameter, which was attached to a collecting glass chamber by a tube. This, in turn, was joined to an electric aspirating pump controlled by Muriel Harris. I quickly steered the needle to the follicle and pierced its wall from the side. 'Right,' I said to Muriel who, under my direction, applied suction. I watched the follicle slowly empty drop by drop into the collecting system. It was beautiful – a slow collapse of the follicle and a clear amber fluid collecting in the glass chamber.

'Stop!' I commanded.

After the chamber was detached from the suction system and a sterile lid placed on it, a nurse carried the precious cargo to the hatch between the theatre and the culture laboratory where Jean received it. She would pass it carefully on to Bob to examine under a microscope, having already put the semen droplets in their dish on the warmed stage. While I waited for Bob's verdict I placed a new glass chamber in position.

'Got it,' I heard Bob say. 'An excellent egg. Just right. I'm happy.'

Bob washed the egg through the culture media using a pipette which he controlled by finger and thumb pressure on a small rubber bulb. I have always admired Bob's skill in using these pipettes. How easily he picked up an egg to transfer it from one droplet to another without losing it – all under microscopic vision.

Now we were working separately. While he was placing the washed egg in a droplet of culture with some 20,000 spermatozoa in it, I, in the operating theatre, was withdrawing the aspirating needle. The diminutive hole in the follicle did not bleed. I took out the cannula and holding forceps. The gas was evacuated and replaced by carbon dioxide. This helped to clear out the other special gas which otherwise would have only been absorbed slowly. Then the carbon dioxide itself was emptied out and the laparoscope withdrawn. Finally I closed the two small incisions with tantalum clips. The operation was over. Within fifteen

minutes of the anaesthetic being started Lesley was awake and
ready to be wheeled back to her bed.

'Did you get an egg?' she asked me softly.

'Yes, a very nice egg. You can go back to sleep.'

Mrs Brown slept for a few hours. At four o'clock that day she
was sitting up happily taking her tea, and later that evening she
was out of bed and walking around a little. It had hardly been a
major ordeal. Meanwhile the egg and the sperms were in the
incubator. By ten o'clock that same night fertilization had
occurred.

Next evening, when I visited Kershaw's again, I examined the
embryo under the microscope. Bob stood to one side after he had
inspected it. It lay on the warm stage with a diffuse light shining
through it from below but I could not see it clearly, for a delicate
tissue surrounded it like a spherical halo. This was derived from
the egg's cumulus which clung to parts of the embryo's surface.
I gently shook the dish and the embryo rolled over. There! I
could see two rounded pale cells filling the original membranes
– the first cleavage having taken place. How extraordinary that
these cells could potentially grow and develop into a baby. The
embryo was returned to the incubator and when I saw Lesley,
who had now fully recovered, I told her about the cleavage of
the cells. She smiled. It seemed she expected nothing less.

Next morning Bob called me. 'The Browns' embryo has now
reached the four-cell stage,' he said. 'Would you please be
available to replace the embryo this evening?'

But it was Friday 12 November, Sheena's birthday. We had
planned a small dinner party at the Normandie restaurant at
Birtle, near Bury. The owners of the restaurant were good friends
of ours. It was an occasion that both Sheena and I had been
looking forward to.

'I'll come at seven, replace the embryo, then go on to Birtle,' I
said.

At seven, Bob told me the embryo was only six-celled, so off
we went to our dinner party. We would have to come back a
little early, that was all, and also I would have to forgo the
celebratory birthday drinks, the wine that the others in our party
would, of course, happily imbibe. At the Normandie my friends
kept telling me how good these wines were while I doggedly
drank vintage English water. As a Chevalier du Tastevin I had
chosen the wines myself and knew the quality of what I was

missing. Soon after ten o'clock we were back at Kershaw's. The embryo stubbornly had still not become eight-celled, so we just had to wait. I recall how the four of us – Bob, Jean, Sheena and I – talked for hours about our earlier years and of our hopes for the future, for women like Lesley Brown. At last we turned to more mundane matters.

'Are you going abroad again soon?' asked Bob, who had told me that he and Ruth would soon be off to Holland.

'Early December I'm going to a laparoscopy meeting in San Francisco,' I replied.

'In March we're both having a holiday in Barbados,' Sheena said, 'partly in a hotel, and partly on a Cunard cruiser!'

Sheena and I longed to return to Barbados, where I had successfully convalesced after my hip operations. I was about to recommend Barbados to all and sundry when Bob stood up. I looked at my watch. It was nearly midnight.

'We'd better have another look,' Bob said.

Bob and Jean examined the embryo once more. At last it had eight cells. I took a brief glimpse at it. It was beautiful: eight rounded, perfect cells. The cumulus cells had broken away and I was filled with awe at the loveliness of this minuscule dot of potential human life. It was time to change into my hospital blues and to move Lesley Brown into the theatre so that I could replace this same vibrant dot into the body of her womb.

As I changed I plunged my face into ice-cold water. Lesley was now in the theatre in position. It was not long before I unveiled the sterile tray that had been previously prepared by Muriel Harris. Bob stood by, gowned and gloved. I put together the little plastic cannula and syringe, then handed it to him. He went to the adjacent lab to load the precious embryo into the end of the cannula under microscopic control. This step required nerves of steel. And while Bob was doing this I covered Lesley with sterile green towels and gently exposed the entrance to her womb.

'Are you comfortable?' I asked Lesley.

'Yes.'

I gently swabbed the cervix with some warm culture fluid – the entrance to it was clean and healthy. Now we waited. Lesley Brown and I waited for Bob and Jean. We had to wait two long minutes. At last Bob was at my side holding the loaded tube and syringe in two hands. I guided the syringe towards the entrance with my left hand and the tube, firmly in the grip of long

dissecting forceps, with my right hand. Forwards and inwards to
the opening into which mercifully the smoothed end of the tube
slid. We held steady. Together Bob and I advanced the precious
load into the body of the womb.

'We're right,' I said to Bob.

Jean was watching anxiously. Bob gently advanced the plunger
so as to expel the embryo from the cannula into the womb. We
hoped that now the tiny droplet carrying the embryo had passed
into the lining folds of the womb. Bob released the syringe and
tube entirely into my care and I held steady for one, two minutes
before slowly, cautiously, withdrawing the tube. Bob hovered
close by, ready to receive the whole apparatus as soon as it was
free. It came out gently. I watched the lips of the cervix close
without any sign of fluid being rejected from it. Bob took the
syringe and tube back to the lab microscope. Jean joined him.
They had to make sure the embryo had left the tube.

'All right, Lesley?'

'Fine.'

She seemed relaxed and confident, and soon Jean's smiling eyes
above her mask and her upraised thumb indicated that all was
well. I removed the instrument, releasing Lesley from her uncomfortable position. We moved her gently from the operating table
to the trolley and then on to her bed where she was tucked up
for the night. As Jean bent over her Mrs Brown remarked, 'That
was a wonderful experience.' It seemed she was sure that now
she really had started her baby. I went back to where Sheena was
waiting for me. It was late. Sheena looked sleepy.

'All well?' she asked.

'Yes,' I said. 'Mrs Brown *feels* pregnant.'

We went home. My car headlights luminously probed the
empty roads of darkness.

Next morning Jean and Bob packed their things and returned
to Cambridge.

21
The Breakthrough
Robert Edwards

Lesley Brown had been the second of the three patients we tested with Hi-Gonavis for the LH surge. Number 1, as has already been said, gave us an egg which began cleaving according to plan. Patrick had more difficulty in collecting Mrs Brown's because of post-operative adhesions when her Fallopian tubes were removed, but he managed in the end, and again I was able to exclaim happily, 'Got it!' as I peered down the microscope.

Alas, we did not have the same success with the third patient. The egg somehow eluded us at laparoscopy. No matter – two out of three bull's-eyes was a bright beginning. We had crossed a barrier, leaving behind us the fertility drugs and their devastating effects on the womb. To me, it meant that we had to be prepared to work all hours of the day and night testing hormones or performing the laparoscopy. The LH surge demanded it. And at least now the wombs of our patients, not having been assaulted by extraneous hormones, should be ready to welcome any embryo introduced into them.

We observed the two embryos we had achieved cleaving in our culture fluids. The first one, several days after fertilization, had divided into eight cells and it was time for it to be implanted in its mother. How carefully that November evening did I draw it into a cannula and walk with it the fifteen paces to the operating theatre where Patrick was waiting. He, in turn, gently inserted the cannula into the womb and afterwards the patient was returned to her bed for the evening. All we could do now was to cross our fingers.

The next morning, when I saw that the second embryo – that of Mr and Mrs Brown – had grown to four cells, I asked Patrick to come over to Kershaw's that evening to replace it in her womb. It was then that I heard about Sheena Steptoe's birthday dinner.

The coincidence of its occurring at the same time as the embryo's slow division into eight cells was to lead to so many developments.

When Patrick and Sheena returned from their restaurant the embryo still had only seven cells, and in the two hours that we waited for that last cell to divide into two we talked and talked about the past and the future, about Oldham and Cambridge, and above all about Patrick's forthcoming retirement. It amazed me – and it still does – that he had not been utterly discouraged by all our failures. It was surprising that he had not become sceptical and tired of my recurring enthusiasms – or, for that matter, of my threats of 'no more' when we had stumbled once again. On the contrary, it was always Patrick who would insist upon continuing our quest. Well, he had patients awaiting our treatment, pressing him, full of their personal tragedies and their whispered longings. He had promises to keep. But now our quest had become a race against the clock, with his retirement scheduled for June 1978. All the same he was still at his peak and certainly not the sort of man to stop working.

At midnight, the embryo we were awaiting consisted at last of eight lovely cells, all even and round, nicely shaped, obviously vibrant with energy. It was time to collect our patient. We left Sheena in the sitting room, still in her evening dress, her birthday over.

Once again I took the embryo in its cannula to Patrick in Kershaw's tiny operating theatre, and watched as he guided it into Mrs Brown's womb, expelled the embryo and then, after a pause, withdrew the cannula. Gently we wheeled our patient to her bed and Jean tucked her in for the night.

Mrs Brown seemed totally relaxed. She said to Jean, 'That was a marvellous experience.' It seemed a strange thing to say. Then she added quietly, 'Thank you very much.'

Next morning she was walking about having experienced no pains in her womb, no contractions that could expel the newly replanted embryo. Jean and I left the ward, returned to the laboratory, washed everything thoroughly and prepared to return to Cambridge. Having replaced the embryos in both the patients we had no reason to stay on at Oldham. Besides, in less than two weeks, Ruth and I were going to a meeting in Holland and I had many things to see to in Cambridge before then. Mr Holmes promised to forward us regular urine and blood samples of the

two patients for our analysis. And that was that. Soon we were
threading our way out of Oldham and driving south.

Just before Ruth and I left for Holland I learnt that our first
patient had begun to menstruate. So our first attempt had failed.
It was curiously disappointing. I knew how Patrick in Kershaw's
would be saying to her in the old disconsolate way, 'We're as
sorry as you are. Come back whenever you want and we'll try
again.' At least, our second patient, Mrs Brown, though two
weeks had passed since we had replaced her embryo, had not yet
manifested any signs of menstruation. We would be in Holland
for only three days and I hoped fervently that we would not be
confronted with more bad news on our return.

On the contrary, when we did arrive back in Cambridge we
learnt that Mrs Brown's period still had not commenced –
eighteen days since the embryo implant! No wonder I began to
examine with increasing eagerness the hormones in the urine
and blood samples that Mr Holmes so diligently sent on to us.
The trouble was that there was a delay between the collecting of
the samples and our results.

No matter. When Jean showed me the most recent result – it
looked very interesting to her – my blood started racing. Wasn't
there a hint of pregnancy, a little blip in that analysis? By now
twenty days had passed since the replacement of the embryo and
Mrs Brown still had not resumed her cycle. The next results
should be crucial. They were. The blip was bigger, more definite.
The following results told the same happy story – the pregnancy
hormones were rising.

'We've done it,' I told Jean excitedly. 'Moreover our patient
has no Fallopian tubes, none whatsoever, so this time it cannot
be an ectopic pregnancy.' I knew, too that Patrick had found a
positive pregnancy test in Oldham.

So, without the fertility drugs, we had managed it at our
second attempt. I wrote a little note to Mrs Brown on 6 December
1977.

'Dear Mrs Brown,' I scribbled. 'Just a short note to let you
know that the early results on your blood and urine samples are
very encouraging and indicate that you might be in early pregnancy. So please take things quietly – no skiing, climbing, or
anything too strenuous including Xmas shopping! If you should
wish to get in touch with me for any reason before seeing Mr
Steptoe next week, my laboratory number is _____ Best

wishes, yours sincerely, R. G. Edwards.'

My threadbare note was hardly a literary masterpiece, yet I heard later that Mrs Brown had read it a hundred times. Patrick, Jean and I were equally delighted. We had given Mrs Brown neither hormones nor drugs; the embryo's growth had been excellent, even to the last division of that recalcitrant cell at midnight. We had made our breakthrough.

Word spread around. In Kershaw's, and in Oldham General Hospital, they were all talking about Mrs Brown's pregnancy. Nurses, cleaners, cooks, along of course with our patients, shared with us the excitement of it all. We all knew, though, that there were some eight months or so to go yet.

I wanted to establish three other pregnancies before we quit Kershaw's. That would prove the efficacy of our methods. We had until August by courtesy of the Area Health Authority although Patrick would be retiring from the National Health Service in June. 'We could continue our work at Manchester,' Patrick had suggested to me. 'Several hospitals have offered me facilities there.' But Jean and I had had enough of travelling north – we had done this for over a decade. No, it would be better to set up something nearer Cambridge and surely, if in the next six months we did have three successful pregnancies, we would be helped to do exactly that. 1978 was going to be a crucial year and as soon as Christmas was over I guessed that Jean and I would become frantically busy.

Indeed the first two weeks of the New Year turned out to be even more hectic than I had expected. We brought sixteen patients into Kershaw's and had to test their urine samples repeatedly to discover when their LH surge began. Apart from the hormone tests we had to continue making our culture fluids, clean and sterilize the rooms, prepare the equipment and apparatus, assist Patrick at the laparoscopy, fertilize the eggs, watch over the cleavage until the embryos were developed to eight cells, then help Patrick with the replacements. No wonder I was often to be found wandering down the corridors of Kershaw's Hospital, unshaven, dog-tired, anxious about this or that hormone result. We did not often get to bed before 1 a.m. And we always rose at 6 a.m. ready to check the hormones again. Jean and I agreed to take turns at slipping downstairs during the hours of darkness to check the Hi-Gonavis. I fondly imagined that our nocturnal tests went unnoticed – that the patients were fast asleep in their beds. They all seemed so peaceful and tranquil and silent. I learnt later that they had all been awake, tensed up, waiting with bated breath for me to come and tell them that their surge had started and their turn was next. They lay in the dark secretly listening for the slight squeak of the sliding door of our tiny laboratory.

It was worth every ounce of our effort. We discovered that our November work was repeatable. The strain though was also considerable upon the operating staff who had to come over to Kershaw's for laparoscopies often just before midnight – and they had already done a day's work at Oldham General and would be undertaking another operating list on the morning of the morrow! The trouble was Nature had designed that our patients' surges often began at awkward times, making night work a routine necessity.

Our methods had to be simplified to subdue some of the pressures upon us. We managed to modify the interval between the surge of LH and the laparoscopy so that the latter was able to take place between 8 a.m. and 9 p.m. We refined our other techniques too. For instance, by using the intercom system between the room where we carried out the cultures and the operating theatre, we could let Patrick know instantly that we had found the ripening egg so that he could end the operation at once. We became so skilled and so organized that, on one occasion, the egg was in the culture fluids within two minutes of Patrick first seeing the ripening follicle. Two minutes of surgery and a chance of pregnancy where there had been none before.

22

The Noise of the Day, the Peace of the Night

Robert Edwards

During January we replaced embryos into nine of our patients. If three or four of these would become pregnant it would bring our work at Kershaw's to a grandstand victorious end. And not only would we have helped those patients who had no Fallopian tubes but also outdated the method that relied on surgical repair of the blocked tubes to gain a pregnancy – the latter operation took two or more hours while ours lasted only some two or more minutes. Alas, we did not do well with those attempted pregnancies that January. Only one of the nine women became pregnant. That in itself was marvellous, confirming that we were on the right lines. But why had we failed with the others? Their menstrual cycles began exactly on time as if they had never received an embryo.

'It's not the embryos – they were excellent,' I said to Jean. 'There may be a better way perhaps of placing them in the uterus. I don't know.'

Back in Cambridge I retired to the libraries to read everything I could find in the journals about embryos, about the womb, about anything that might be relevant – whether in monkeys, cows, rats, mice or hamsters. At last I thought I had found a clue. The womb can produce chemicals that cause it to contract. Supposing a small contraction occurred immediately we had reimplanted the embryo? Why, this might cause it to be expelled, so undoing everything we had planned and fought for. There were one or two antidotes including aspirin. Aspirin prevents the formation of the chemical that produces the uterine contraction and alleviates its effect.

'We'll give our patients aspirin,' I said to Jean, 'when we replace their embryos. Just before and just after.'

It was a long shot but worth a try. The results were disastrous. We observed with dismay how our patients' hormones subsided

and declined before menstruation began. We gained no pregnancies at all. Our only consolation was that the two pregnant
patients were well and progressing normally. In Mrs Brown's
case we knew that she was carrying a baby daughter and that all
the tests on the baby's chromosomes had proved to be most
satisfactory.

It was back to the Cambridge library for me to read, read, read.
Suddenly a glimmer of an idea came when, in two recent separate
papers, I stumbled on reports describing a pronounced daily
rhythm in the hormones of female rats and of female monkeys
soon after ovulation. The hormone changes typical of early
pregnancy did not apparently rise steadily but fluctuated during
the day: they were low in the morning, high in the evening. I
was deeply familiar with other daily cycles – every scientist and
doctor working in reproductive biology knows of them. But this
pronounced daily cycle I knew nothing of. It was new to me.
Why, I thought, *if these hormones are highest in the evening
and lowest in the morning then we should be replacing our
embryos at night when the hormones are highest.* Another reason
occurred to me for replacing the embryos at night. The adrenal
gland that controls day-to-day activity is itself least active at
night. Wouldn't it be sensible therefore to replace embryos when
all is peaceful in the evening for that reason too? I read and re-
read these reports as well as several other papers on the same
subject. The more I thought about it the more I felt that the very
time of inserting the embryo into the womb could be a most
significant matter.

I recalled the evening we replaced the embryo into Mrs Brown.
Had we not talked, all of us, until midnight while waiting for
the embryo to move to its eight-celled stage? That successful
pregnancy had begun at dead of night. And when I checked on
the timing in our second pregnancy, I learnt with excitement
that that embryo had also been replaced in the evening. What
about those pregnancies that occurred when we had used the
fertility drugs and HCG? The patient with the ectopic pregnancy
and the two other women with abortive ones according to our
records, had also had their embryos replaced after 5 p.m. All our
morning efforts had failed. Almost all the failures since New
Year's Day had replants done between breakfast and lunch. The
adrenal hormones must have been high when the embryos had
been replaced and, if what was true for rats and monkeys was

also true for women, the ovarian hormones had been low.

Were my deductions correct? It was May. We had so little time left at Kershaw's. At this late date I began to think the embryos might even implant normally during the evening, two or three days after they first entered the womb – either naturally or after artificial replacement. But supposing there were other reasons for our success when embryos were replaced at night rather than during the day? One morning at Kershaw's I stood still and listened. I heard noisy vacuum cleaners, trolleys rattling, people distinctly talking, doctors and nurses bustling in and out of rooms; in short, a small cacophony of noises – a modern symphony, if you like, to jangle the nerves of anxious waiting patients and stimulate their adrenal glands to pour out hormones into the bloodstream. At night, when I stood at the same spot, it was so serenely quiet and still that I could hear someone clear his throat, then only the faint footsteps of a nurse on her rounds. I thought it most likely that the daily cycle of the womb was the main factor but there was just a chance, of course, that our successes and failures could be related to the hospital's cyclic bustle of events or, for that matter, to my own cycle or Patrick's or Jean's.

In any event we decided to replace the embryo into the wombs of our next five patients at Kershaw's late in the evening. Once again urine collections every three hours, assays for oestrogen and LH, night and day, in order to give warnings to Patrick and his team. Once again, eventually, the evening peace and quiet of Kershaw's was shattered as they arrived to invade the tiny operating theatre for the laparoscopy. Patrick would usually arrive first. The doors of Kershaw's would suddenly be flung open and in would storm Patrick, walking briskly despite his artificial hips. Soon after, his perspiring registrar would push through the same doors, trying to keep up as he rushed to the changing room and donned his hospital blues. Three minutes later a bevy of nurses would arrive, in their midst Dr Mukherjee and the anaesthetist from the Oldham General. How quickly the team would assemble, the theatre be ready, the patient wheeled in. Ten minutes later they would all be leaving, the anaesthetist for his home, then Patrick and the other doctors and finally the nurses. It would be quiet again.

We replaced embryos into four of our patients during the evening – the other, for reasons beyond our control, in the morning. The embryos were a day older this time than previously – they were sixteen-celled. After the reimplantations Mr Holmes, as usual, collected samples of urine and blood for us to analyse the hormones and to keep watch over the progress of our patients towards either menstruation or pregnancy. To our delight one of the four evening reimplantations began to display all the signs of pregnancy. The patient's hormones continued to rise slowly and steadily. So we had three pregnancies now. We had every reason to feel buoyant. Suddenly, though, we had cause for anxiety: Mrs Brown displayed the early signs of toxaemia of pregnancy.

'Her blood pressure is a little raised,' said Patrick, alarmed, 'but there is no albumen in the urine.'

The growth of the baby was slower than expected. It was Mrs Brown's thirtieth week of pregnancy. How sickening, how tragic, if anything went awry now! To complicate matters further the press had, with a vengeance, discovered Lesley Brown. It was hardly surprising. Her regular journeys from her home in Bristol to Oldham for consultations with Patrick had not gone unnoticed. All the staff at Oldham General Hospital and Kershaw's – the nurses, the secretaries, the cleaners, the administrators knew of the successful pregnancy and gossiped about it. So, too, did hundreds of infertile patients for whom Mrs Brown had become a symbol of hope.

No one inexperienced in the pressures of the press can appreciate the stress and trauma of it. Reporters began to circle the hospital grounds with long-range cameras, long-range recorders, every modern device of intrusion. They began interfering at Kershaw's too – names of past and present patients being printed. Some member of the hospital staff obviously was giving away confidential information about patients, had stolen names and addresses from hospital records along with reports on Mrs Brown's health and progress at Kershaw's. Money talked. They were offering £5000 for ten names and addresses of our patients, a further £5000 should any of these ten become a story. A piece of information about Mrs Brown could fetch £1000. Even a telephone number could be worth £300.

This was the situation as Patrick fought to save Lesley Brown's pregnancy, looked after other pregnancies – and as I tried for one more pregnancy at Kershaw's before we left that hospital forever. I watched with fascination as Patrick used all his skill to help Mrs Brown in the final stages of her pregnancy and all his cunning to protect her privacy. It was far from certain that he and Mrs Brown would win through. I have seldom admired Patrick so much as during the next month. When I managed to return briefly to Cambridge I said to Ruth – 'What's happening up there is both marvellous and tragic. We just have to rely on Patrick'.

23
The Delilah of the Press
Patrick Steptoe

When I went off to the meeting about laparoscopy in San Francisco I knew that Lesley Brown was pregnant. Months later, I was chided by friends who had been at that conference. They complained that I had not confided in them about our breakthrough. Of course I would not whisper a word to others about our good news. Bob and I always hoped to report our successes first in the established medical journals. Doctors have always been wary of the popular press. In the last century, Sir William Osler justly wrote: 'In the life of every successful physician there comes the temptation to toy with the Delilah of the press – daily and otherwise. There are times when she may be courted with satisfaction, but beware, sooner or later she is sure to play the harlot, and has left many a man shorn of his strength.'

Both Bob and I believed that the public should be informed about medical advances in a way that could be readily understood. There would be time for that. But not now. There was the privacy of all our patients to consider – not only the privacy of the Browns. The fewer who knew about Lesley's pregnancy, we decided, the better.

It was a forlorn hope. Inevitably patients and staff at Oldham General Hospital and at Kershaw's spoke of Lesley's pregnancy and soon reporters from the local evening newspaper began to poke around relentlessly, intrusively. Meanwhile, Lesley came from Bristol to Oldham for her first ultrasonic scan. This showed a single foetus in the uterus, twelve weeks in size and with a heartbeat present. A month later, not long before our planned holiday in the Caribbean, a second scan showed us the position of the afterbirth and I obtained without difficulty ten millilitres of fluid. The fluid would inform us, we hoped, of the normality of Lesley's baby. I sent it off to the Regional Genetics Department

at St Mary's Hospital in Manchester. Before we left for Barbados
I had already heard from them that the foetus had no neural
defects such as spina bifida or hydrocephalus. I would have to
wait some three weeks more, though, for the chromosome report.
I said to my hospital secretary, Diana Mann, 'If the results of the
chromosome analysis arrive while we are still away, please cable
me.'

On 14 March Sheena and I sat at dinner on board the *Cunard
Countess*. On the table lay a cable which read: 'REPORT AS
REQUESTED STOP FEMALE KARYOTYPE 46XX STOP NO
ABNORMALITY DETECTED STOP R.G.E. INFORMED STOP
DIANA.'

We ordered a bottle of champagne and raised our glasses to
the health and happiness of John and Lesley Brown and to the
future of Miss Brown.

'Will you tell Lesley she's going to have a daughter?' Sheena
asked.

'No, I don't think so,' I replied.

We informed the Browns about the result of the test but
not of the sex of the foetus. That the test was normal came as
a huge relief to them. After all their longings for a child, it
would have been a cruel blow if they'd had, at this stage, to
have the pregnancy terminated. For them, this last, almost
unspoken, anxiety dissolved utterly. They believed that, supported by their families, they could now settle down quietly
for a normal and happy pregnancy. How wrong that belief
turned out to be.

It was a wonderful feeling to be so confident about our new
approach. Despite the extra work, the inconvenience, I wished
we had dispensed with the fertility drugs earlier. For now,
when I spoke to this or that patient – though of course I had
to be guarded about promising certain fulfilment of a long-
frustrated desire for a baby – I could afford to be somewhat
optimistic. We had two pregnancies both proceeding normally.
It seemed likely that we would have more.

Bob Edwards really was an extraordinary man. When one
of his ideas came to nothing he would not be downcast too
long. Soon, enthusiastically, he would be presenting us with
another idea. Now he was suggesting that we might obtain a
greater rate of success with our patients if we gave them
aspirin just before and just after replacing an embryo into the

uterus. The aspirin was an antidote to any possible small
uterine contractions that the procedure triggered off.

It was worth a try. We brought more patients into Kershaw's. Once again I was busy working with Bob and Jean,
sometimes in the morning, sometimes in the evening, whenever the circumstances dictated. One night I returned home
dog-tired from Kershaw's and sank into an armchair. Almost
at once the telephone rang. A few moments later Sheena said,
'It's New York.' Sighing, I rose.

'Is it true,' a lady with an American accent was asking, 'that
you and Dr Edwards have gained several successful pregnancies following embryo replacements?'

'Who is this?' I asked.

'The *New York Post*,' the woman said.

I assumed that the *New York Post* reporter was referring to
those three previous pregnancies that had failed and which
we had already reported. 'What about other pregnancies?' my
inquisitor insisted. 'Have you any *on-going* pregnancies at the
present time?' I hesitated.

'Any progress in our work will be conveyed to our medical
and scientific colleagues through the proper orthodox channels,' I said coldly and put down the phone as soon as I
decently could.

No use. Next day the New York paper published that we
had 'on-going pregnancies'. This proved too much for our local
Oldham newspaper. On 20 April they declared that the world's
first test-tube baby would be born in Oldham in July. They
reported – quite untruthfully – that sums in excess of £100,000
had been offered for the exclusive rights of the story.

Usually Lesley Brown spent most of her day alone at home
in Bristol while her husband was at work. Suddenly she was
confronted at the front and back doors by ill-informed and
often unscrupulous roving reporters. John also began to be
pestered daily to and from work. It became impossible. The
truth is the Browns never sought publicity and wished to be
alone. When Lesley reacted under the stress of these hounding
intrusions I arranged for her to rest a while at my daughter's
house in Suffolk. Afterwards, it was no longer possible for her
to return home. Reporters were waiting and watching outside
her house. Instead she joined relatives who lived elsewhere in
Bristol and Dr Hinton cleverly arranged for Lesley to have

continuing medical attention.

A number of reporters may have trailed around Bristol in search of Lesley but it seemed to me that the rest of the world's press descended on Oldham. There were journalists from newspapers, from magazines, from television and radio, and we were compelled to ask our administrators for security measures to keep out a number of these nosy reporters and photographers who were trespassing into Kershaw's. Our other patients there needed protection. Lesley's whereabouts were kept remarkably secret during May and, in June, I drove her myself from Bristol to Oldham – for I was now determined that she should be under my personal care during the last eight weeks of her pregnancy. Lesley was admitted to our maternity block at Oldham on Sunday, 11 June thirty-two weeks and three days pregnant, under an assumed name. Only two members of the staff knew who she really was.

The growth of the baby was laggard. I was worried. Our long vigil began. It was most important that we should watch for any increasing signs of placental insufficiency since this would indicate danger to the foetus in the womb.

'If the baby gets to weigh more than five pounds eight ounces with mature healthy tissue – particularly of lungs and liver,' I explained to Sheena, 'that should be OK.'

Another of our patients had become pregnant and I should have been jubilant, but I was concerned for Mrs Brown and Mrs Brown's baby. On 21 June when Lesley was thirty-four weeks pregnant ultrasonic measurements of the foetus indicated a size corresponding only to thirty weeks. A week later the growth still lagged behind, and now Lesley developed a mild but persistent toxaemia of pregnancy. Toxaemia occurs in about 10 per cent of all pregnancies. How unfortunate that this should happen to Lesley. A toxaemia meant that at any time her condition could deteriorate quickly, either by a rapid rise of blood pressure or by a lowering of kidney function with retention of fluids in the body. Such worsening of the toxaemia could cause death of the baby while still in the womb, or a serious haemorrhage from the placenta inside, which could threaten both mother and baby. It would be best for the baby to be out of the womb but it was not yet big enough. I would have to watch Lesley's condition very carefully indeed.

Meanwhile journalistic offences and misrepresentations

abounded. None of my patients was safe from invasion of
their privacy. Even ex-patients who had left Kershaw's were
subjected to impertinent enquiries. One day a phone call had
me rushing over to Lesley. 'She's in a state,' I was told. No
wonder. She had read in a local paper sensational speculations
about the possible death of her baby. She was in tears. 'It said
that my baby nearly died yesterday,' she sobbed. 'Is it true?
Will it happen again?'
   'No, no,' I said. 'It isn't true. All is well.'
   I examined her. Her blood pressure was further raised as a
result of these anxieties and when I listened to the heartbeat
of the foetus in her abdomen it was disturbed. I set about to
calm her and sedate her. When I left I felt angry – angry at
gutter journalism. The newspaper's speculative report had
been based on information given them by one of their hospital
spies. Confidential hospital reports had been stolen and presented in this sensational way. I was angry with the reporter
who had upset Lesley. John was furious. If he could have
identified him he would have bloodied his nose.
   After my anger cooled down, I felt sad. Over the years we
had built up a team of doctors, nurses, midwives, secretaries,
technicians, domestics and porters who respected and trusted
each other, who treated each other with professional affection.
Now each was suspicious of the other. Who was destroying
this rapport, and what were the authorities, including the top
administrators of the Health Service, doing about it? Instead of
June and July being happy months for us they were constantly
marred by interference. A local detective agency busied itself
trying to bribe and cajole members of the staff into giving
away confidential secrets. Was anything being done by the
administrators to remedy the situation? Pressmen were circling
the hospital, trying to gain entrance by any means. They
dressed up as boilermakers, plumbers, window cleaners, but
the hospital administrators felt unable to protect Mrs Brown
by posting guards on her door and keeping out intruders. They
maintained it was not the function of the National Health
Service to provide protection of patients in this way. I wrote a
letter to the *British Medical Journal* and complained to the
Secretary and to the Chairman of the Manchester Regional
Health Authority.
   The last three weeks of Lesley's pregnancy became partic-

ularly trying. Her toxaemia was persistent. I found alarming
variations from time to time in the foetal heart rate. I spent
more and more time at the hospital. At least the baby's growth
progressed and indeed it began to catch up. But one ghastly
evening Edwin Warren, the Area Administrator, contacted
me. 'There's a bomb scare,' he said sombrely.
  'What?'
  'Someone has telephoned to say that a bomb has been placed
in the maternity building.'
  'You're joking.'
  'No. We have to act,' he replied. 'So I have called in the
police.'
  Was this an effort to smoke out Lesley Brown? Every patient
had to be evacuated to nearby wards along with their babies.
Women in labour had to be moved too, and also those women
recovering from operations performed that very day. Within
thirty minutes the building was empty and trained police dogs
were taken in to sniff out any possible explosives. It took two
hours for the Oldham police to declare the building safe. They
did a marvellous job.
  The pressure on the Browns had been alleviated to some
extent when they entered into a modest contract with one
newspaper group for *their* story. We respected their right to
do this, especially as by now they could in no way escape the
publicity; besides it seemed wise that they should do some
thing to help the child's future. Bob and I too were offered
enormous sums for exclusive stories but the conditions
required were quite unacceptable to us. The newspaper group
had provided burly security guards for Lesley and this action
provoked the hospital authorities, somewhat belatedly, to take
over security and, at last, to stop intruders getting into Lesley's
room.
  But even these measures did not help me to sleep well at
night. I worried about Lesley. Would her blood pressure shoot
up suddenly? Would the foetal heart stop? Just imagine the
kind of publicity – apart from the Browns' grief – if such a
thing happened. I was not sleeping at all well.
  Happily the foetal heart continued to beat, Lesley's blood
pressure did not increase and, much to my relief, the baby's
growth suddenly spurted. Sometimes it's a help to talk to a
respected colleague. On the week-end of 22 July I discussed all

the medical details of the case with Professor Tindall of St
Mary's Hospital, Manchester, and in so doing I clarified for
myself the various courses of action I would need to take in
the face of various possible contingencies.

Monday was pandemonium day at Oldham. A press information office had been set up with desks and telephones. The
Minister of Health, the Central Office of Information and the
Regional Officers had together advised Bob and me to hold a
press conference and to give television interviews within
hours of the birth. The Central Office of Information had been
given the job of sending up a unit to film the birth if the
Browns agreed. The birth, after all, would be an historic
occasion. We wanted it filmed. We wanted a government
organization, the Central Office of Information, to do all the
filming. Then, when they sold the film to the highest bidder,
the proceeds could be given to the National Health Service.
The NHS should have some credit and so should the Oldham
and the North West Regional Health authorities for all the
help that they had given us over the years. But now everybody
seemed to be arguing with everybody else, and to be asking
my opinion about it all.

As for the real matter in hand I knew by the end of the day
that the morrow would be the day of decision. Much depended
on the results of numerous tests. Would Lesley continue her
pregnancy or should she be delivered? They were still arguing
when I quit the hospital: who had the right to do what, who
owned the copyrights – the hospital, the Browns, or the
Department of Health and Social Security? I drove home
exhausted. It was late. I lay awake in bed for what seemed
hours before falling into a fitful sleep.

24
Day of Decision
Patrick Steptoe

It was the fifth day in the thirty-ninth week of Lesley Brown's pregnancy, Tuesday 25 July, a dull, close, cloudy day with only occasional glimpses of the sun. The programme at Kershaw's hung fire and Bob had taken the opportunity to relax at his cottage in Yorkshire, leaving Jean to hold the fort and look at some of the assays as they came through.

My morning was taken up with further assessments of Lesley's toxaemia and I decided that the *liquor amnii*, the precious fluid in the sac surrounding Lesley's baby, should be examined. The fluid was obtained at noon with the skilled assistance of Dr Collighan, one of our radiologists, who carried out an ultrasonic scan, and it was rushed by taxi to that great maternity teaching hospital, St Mary's, Manchester.

I waited impatiently for the results as I spent the afternoon seeing a stream of patients. There was one item of extremely good news. When Dr Collighan made his ultrasonic scan to find where the pool of liquor lay in the uterus, he had also used his 'echo-sounding' machine to measure the size of the foetal head. To our delight, it had at last reached a diameter of 9.6 centimetres, corresponding to a baby maturity of thirty-eight weeks.

That measurement of growth had been lagging behind the dates of the pregnancy for several weeks. When Lesley was thirty-five weeks pregnant the head measurement indicated only a thirty-one-week size; at thirty-six weeks only thirty-two; at thirty-seven only thirty-three. But after a sudden glorious spurt of growth at thirty-eight weeks it was thirty-five and now, at thirty-eight weeks and five days, thirty-eight weeks exactly.

At 4.45 p.m. the telephone rang on my office desk. 'There's a Dr Hill on the line,' said my secretary. 'Will you speak to him?'

I knew the moment of decision was at hand. 'Yes, please put

him through.' I had never met Dr Hill but I welcomed his disembodied voice speaking from the biochemistry department at St Mary's.

'The ratio is 3.9 to one,' Dr Hill said cheerfully.

I had to be certain. 'Are you sure? 3.9 to one?'

'Yes, of course.'

'Thank you very much. I'm very grateful to you for ringing me so quickly.

'Not at all. You must be very pleased.'

I was. The figure Dr Hill had just given me was the lecithin–sphingomyelin (LS) ratio in the *liquor amnii*. Provided the ratio was at least 2 to 1 or higher, the baby could be born safely. This ratio of 3.9 to 1 confirmed the baby's maturity, not only by size but by its capacity to breathe well at birth. It meant that the lungs, so small and collapsed, would expand at once, vitally and vigorously with the first respiratory efforts at birth. The quality of that first breath is so important.

So, at 5.00 p.m. on that Tuesday, I knew I could deliver the baby and that its size and weight would be above the level usually described as premature. I was relieved. The toxaemia from which Lesley had been suffering for the last three weeks was under some measure of control; but it would be best if the baby was out of the womb and beginning an independent life. For this to occur Lesley could either have labour induced or she could be delivered by Caesarean section. The normal course of labour introduces certain risks to the child which can be negligible in normal deliveries but quite serious if added to the risks arising from toxaemia. On the other hand a Caesarean section could avoid the long and possibly drawn-out hazards of an induced delivery.

One mile away from my office, the grounds of Oldham General Hospital were patrolled by scouting reporters from the media, awaiting developments. How was I to alert everyone concerned that we were now ready to deliver, without alerting the reporters? I wished to avoid starting things in motion before the night staff reported for duty. It would be much easier to control the hospital grounds and buildings once the usual evening visitors had left. It would not be too complicated to organize the anaesthetist, the paediatricians, the nursing staff, the operating theatres in a short time, but the problem was how to prepare Lesley. She had to be starved for about 8 hours so that her stomach would be empty at the time of starting the anaesthetic.

A little gentle subterfuge was indicated. Edith Marshall, night supervisor of the midwifery staff in the maternity block had made great friends with Lesley, and they respected and trusted each other. By sheer luck, Edith was off duty and in my office at that very moment, helping me out during the absence of one of my usual team on holiday. I took her aside.

'Edith, would you please go to Lesley's room at the hospital right away as if it was one of your usual visits. Tell her confidentially not to eat or drink anything from the moment you see her. We won't alert the rest of the hospital staff just yet. Not even John. Please tell her that I'll be along soon to explain everything.'

Edith drove off in her little car. I knew I could trust her implicitly. I had known her for twenty years, when she first joined us as a student nurse.

I saw my last two patients in a relatively unhurried fashion. As I drove to the hospital the sun came out and with splashes of colour lit up the yellow stone of the new buildings in the town centre, softening the dirty derelict spaces which had been cleared of their old tenements in preparation for the new by-pass extension. Parking the car at the hospital presented the usual problems. It was never too easy to avoid the dug-out holes in the main drive and find a space, but there, near the children's ward, I spotted my wife's car. 'Good, she must be visiting Lesley,' I thought. Sheena, with her warm sympathy towards people with problems, had developed a rapport with both John and Lesley Brown. I hurried past the enquiring marauders with a smile and without comment. It was my custom to visit the wards about this time.

The security guards at the entrance reassured me with a friendly greeting that all was fairly quiet, and on the ward floor further guards were in their customary position outside the delivery area, which was separated from the rest of the lying-in wards by a pair of double doors.

As I entered Lesley's fairly large and light room with its own bathroom and lavatory, I heard the chuckles of two conspirators. The doorway was guarded by a large screen inside, so that no invading photographer could steal a quick photograph without permission from Lesley. I rounded the screen and there was Sheena stuffing the last of Lesley's supper into a polythene bag and then into a shopping basket. The supper tray was remarkably

clean of all food, and the teacup empty. The tea had disappeared
down the washbasin.

The ward sister bustled in. 'Would you like some more tea?
You *have* eaten well. Are you still hungry?'

'No, thank you. I have had quite enough.'

Sister departed, and the tray was removed. I checked the charts,
Lesley's blood pressure, her urinary output, and then felt her
tummy. The baby's head was entering the pelvis and I could
hear the foetal heart beating loud and clear at a rate of 148 beats
per minute. On many occasions during the last two weeks it had
reached high rates, even as high as 180 beats. This was hard to
understand. There was a possibility, I surmised, of something
unusual about the umbilical cord leading to occasional lack of
oxygen for the baby. All other features of the heart rate seemed
normal and there were no sinister decelerations.

'Lesley,' I told her, 'your baby is ready to be born. Because of
all the circumstances I'd like to deliver it tonight by an operation.'

'Whatever you think best. At what time?'

'You won't be ready until eleven o'clock at the earliest. Just
have your visitors as usual, don't let anyone suspect anything,
and let John go home at his usual time of 9.00 p.m. I'll call him
back at the right moment. Make sure you don't have anything
more to eat and drink, and I'll tell John all about it. I'm going
home now but I'll see you later. Sheena will come back again
and stay with John, here, during the operation.'

I saw Sheena to her car with her loaded basket, and then I
went to the office of Fred Baxter, the Sector Administrator, near
the hospital entrance, where an endless argument was going on
among different groups about who had what rights to film the
birth of the baby. The hospital authorities had been besieged for
many days by numerous commercial television film companies
from every part of the world. All had been denied. Finally, when
it was almost too late, the Department of Health and Social
Security had decided to send a film crew. I was introduced to the
film director of this unit from the Central Office of Information.
I explained to him that we could only allow a three-man team
into the operating theatre for camera, lights and sound, so that
there would be no interference with the delivery and the reception of the baby. He told me that his crew would require forty-
five minutes to set up their equipment but that a firm written
contract had still not been agreed and signed by the Regional

Health Authority, the Brown family, represented by a solicitor and himself on behalf of the DHSS. I left them to get on with their negotiations.

As I drove home I realized that my patience was almost at an end. The authorities had known about this impending birth for many weeks, but had apparently given little thought to its impact until the very last moment. World interest had now reached gigantic proportions.

Bob Edwards and I had to remind everybody constantly that the main object was to secure a normal happy mother with a living healthy baby, and that everything else was to remain subservient to this aim. Bob was most anxious that I should be spared as much stress as possible during the last anxious days but he could do little to help, and he was not expected to return to Oldham from his isolated cottage in Yorkshire until eight o'clock that evening. I had been much relieved by discussions on the management of the case with Vic Tindall on the previous Saturday. Our views on the clinical situation were exactly the same. Nevertheless an unpleasant headache was now nagging me and I was glad to reach home and relax for ten minutes at the piano.

Sheena and I drove back to the hospital together, arriving about eight o'clock. We entered surreptitiously by a side door. Nobody noticed us among the busy traffic of hospital visitors now at its peak. Sheena joined Lesley and John Brown while I went to the operating theatre to meet Dr John Webster, who was to assist me at the operation, and Edith Astell who had been my chief scrub-up nurse for several years. She was one of the magnificent team of operating theatre staff trained by Muriel Harris. Sadly, on this important day, Muriel herself was returning from a long-needed holiday in Cornwall and was unable to arrive in time for the actual delivery.

Edith Astell was on duty in charge of the operating suite, and I asked her to be prepared for the Caesarean operation to start at 11.30 p.m. John Webster and I then set off to make all the detailed arrangements from the seclusion of his house just outside the hospital grounds. First, we needed to talk to Bob Edwards who had now returned and to let him and Jean know of the day's events. Then we had to check with Edith Marshall who was on voluntary duty, about Lesley's current condition, and to tell her of the scheduled time of the operation so that she could complete all the preparations.

A telephone call prompted Dr Finlay Campbell, our senior anaesthetist, who agreed to be ready at 11.30 p.m. He had already assessed Lesley for anaesthesia and she needed only an injection of atropine intravenously just before the anaesthetic was started in order to dry up excessive secretions from her respiratory organs. Lastly, I talked to Dr Don Hilson, the paediatrician who was going to be in charge of the reception of the baby, and who, together with his colleagues and assistants, would monitor the first seconds of life and the subsequent progress and care of the infant.

John Brown departed to his temporary home some six miles away and the whole hospital settled quietly into its night routine. Everyone, that is, except the telephone operators! When I went back to the executive offices I found that the wires to London were really hotting up. Discussions were *still* going on between the Minister of Health and the Regional Authority group about the filming. We had already agreed that the news of the birth of the baby would be announced immediately afterwards to everyone through the Press Association, but the question of films and photographs was still controversial and delicate. Bob and I had also agreed that within a few hours of the birth we would give television interviews to both the BBC and ITV channels, and that we would then attend a press conference to be held in Prestwich Hospital, where the correspondents would be provided with numerous telephone lines, not to mention their usual libations!

At 10.30 p.m. I had a little sly enjoyment when I announced to the film manager that he had better get his equipment into the theatre at once. 'A flurried gasp of surprise greeted my words. The group was waiting for copies of the contractual agreement to be typed, and after they arrived more telephone conversations took place with Whitehall about the exact words and phrases. At eleven o'clock, at the end of my patience, I said, with Bob Edwards at my side, that unless everything was tied up in five minutes there would be no film. It is the surgeon's privilege and right that, once an operation starts, he is in absolute charge of everything that goes on in the operating room. His authority is absolute as to who can be admitted and what can go on there. Naturally he guards his patient's interests. He obtains consent before starting to do whatever he considers necessary in the light of the medical circumstances. This authority carries with it a responsibility which we have been trained to accept and exercise in a proper ethical manner.

The sector administrator now decided to increase the security by calling in the help of the Oldham police, who cleared the photographers some distance away from the windows of the corridors, and kept the route from the maternity ward to the theatre tightly controlled.

Within two minutes of my ultimatum all the documents were signed, amidst sighs of relief. I had already arranged for John Brown to be called back to the hospital in time to see Lesley before she was wheeled from the maternity wing to our main operating theatres. Bob, Jean and I made our way there between the rows of policemen to be met by all the rest of the team. We all changed into theatre suits.

At 11.30 p.m. Lesley was wheeled into the anaesthetic room. Bob, Jean and I gathered in a little knot, wished each other luck and went our ways: they, into their masked positions in the theatre, and I to Lesley.

We were alone for a few minutes. I took her hand and comforted her and she smiled. I think we both made our prayers in our own ways at that moment. I listened one last time to the foetal heart. Fifteen seconds noted on the clock, thirty-eight beats counted loud and regular. 152 beats per minute.

I nodded to Finlay, checked that everyone was ready and proceeded to the scrub-up area. I turned on the taps and started to wash. We had done all we possibly could to bring off this event. Of that I was confident. All the tests for normality had been done; no step had been reckless or hurried in all those long struggles. The moment we had all awaited so long was at hand.

25
Birth of a Baby
Patrick Steptoe

In the anaesthetic room, at 11.31 p.m., Finlay Campbell, the anaesthetist, skilfully slid a 'butterfly' needle into a vein on the back of Lesley's hand. A shot of atropine was injected to dry up any excess respiratory secretions, followed by a pentothal solution to induce unconsciousness. Next, a cocktail of muscle relaxants was put into the bloodstream. The bright light of a laryngoscope quickly identified the vocal cords and the trachea, the main tube to the lungs. A long curved rubber tube was passed into it, and a seal was made by means of an inflatable cuff incorporated around the tube, which itself was connected to the anaesthetic machine. Automatic controlled respiration was quickly established, using oxygen mixed with nitrous oxide gas. While this was going on the anaesthetic nurse and the technicians were applying cardiac monitoring equipment, electrical leads were attached to enable the heart to be monitored throughout the operation, and a plate was provided for electrical coagulating forceps to be used by the surgeon to control bleeding points. A plastic sac containing saline solution was inverted and connected to the needle feeding the vein at the back of Lesley's hand. A little later the saline solution would be replaced by blood.

At 11.38 Lesley was wheeled into the operating theatre and lifted from the trolley on to the table, without disturbing any of the vital tubes entering her body. Bright lights had already been switched on and the cinecamera recorded every important move as she was placed carefully in position.

As soon as Finlay was satisfied, the operating team closed round the table. The operating light spilled a bright ring of shadowless intensity on to the bared abdominal wall. This was quickly prepared with cleansing solutions, and sterile green towels were placed over the whole table except for the small clear area where the incision would be made. Instruments were wheeled close in and the vital suction tubes were prepared, one to clear the operating field, and the other, small but very efficient, to clear out the baby's mouth, throat and nose as soon as the delivery of the head allowed.

I stood on the patient's right side, John Webster and Edith Astell opposite. To my right Edith Marshall, scrubbed, gowned and gloved like the rest of us, stood ready to receive the baby. Jennifer Thompson was the 'clean' theatre nurse who prepared all the instrument trolleys and who would be ready to bring any extra or replacement tools which might be required. Don Hilson and the rest of the paediatric team were ready with their resuscitation trolley and special cot which might be needed to help the baby. A nod from the anaesthetist to me, and we started.

I was now totally involved in the technical details of the operation. I had already decided on a vertical incision from the navel to the pubic bone because this gave most room to gain access speedily to the area of womb we wanted.

11.42. Left hand to stretch the skin, right hand to make the scalpel cut through skin and fat down to the muscle layer. Two or three medium vessels spouted blood at the lower end of the incision, and these were quickly sealed with the electric coagulating forceps. I incised the muscle sheath with knife and scissors. At this point, now as always, I remembered with gratitude the trick which my old teacher, David Gwillim, of St George's Hospital, had taught me – how to cut not only forward along a line but backwards by reversing the scissors in the hand, thereby avoiding any clumsy contortions of the surgeon's body.

Now I picked up and incised the peritoneal sac lining the abdominal cavity. There, immediately below, was the bluish pink womb full of baby and fluid. Its lower part was covered by the empty bladder within its protecting sheath which joined on to the womb. The forceps picked up the shining membrane at the join, and my scissors separated bladder and womb along it. Now only the loose tissue between bladder and womb separated me from the part called the lower segment. Gently I pushed the bladder clear, downwards, beneath a shining metal retractor.

The lower segment was thinner than the rest of the womb. Normally it stretches and thins even more during labour 'pains' while the thick muscular upper part of the womb actively contracts to push the baby out of the birth passage and into the world. But this baby was to be spared the stresses of normal labour because of its vulnerability due to the added toxaemia. Caesarean section is only needed for a small number of such cases, unless there are other factors, such as retardation of growth, irregular heart action or other signs of stress. So now I was ready to incise across the thin lower segment, rather like creating a mail-box opening.

The first inch-long incision allowed the thin membranes holding the liquor around the baby to bulge outwards, and my fingers enlarged the transverse opening until it was big enough to accommodate the baby's head. A nick in the bulging membrane, and immediately the whole operation area was flooded with 'milky' liquor. Suction and large swabs to the rescue. My right hand explored into the opening with the membraneous sac downwards into the pelvic basin. I felt the head and slid my fingers easily beyond and below it. A firm hoist and out came the head through the 'letter-box' opening. Baby's face was looking upwards and towards me and the back of the neck was to the mother's left and back.

John Webster wiped away any remaining fluid and sister slipped the suction tube into the baby's mouth. My fingers felt round the neck – no cord wrapped round it, thank goodness. Now John grasped the upper part of Lesley's tummy and pushed down at my direction. The shoulders appeared in the wound followed quickly by the trunk as I lifted and supported the baby along the back with my right arm and forearm. Left hand under the buttocks and out she came. 11.47 p.m.

Glorious. She was chubby, full of muscular tone. The cord was pulsating strongly although it was hooked round the left thigh. I held the head low and we sucked and cleared the mouth and throat. She took a deep breath. Then she yelled and yelled and yelled. I laid her down, all pink and furious, and saw at once that she was externally perfect and beautiful. One minute after the birth the cord stopped pulsating and we clamped it, divided it, and handed the baby to Edith Marshall.

The new citizen continued to cry very loudly, and how we all loved that wonderful sound. She was wrapped and placed head low in a cot, and once more the throat and mouth were cleared of any possible remaining fluid so that she could only inhale good clean air. Don Hilson examined her minutely whilst I was removing the afterbirth from the upper part of the womb. This was handed over to the other paediatricians who measured the cord length, took some cord blood for tests, and weighed the afterbirth. Meanwhile, I was rapidly closing up the letter-box in the womb with two rows of stitches, and then replacing the bladder with a light suture along its former joint. We cleaned out all the fluid and blood which had spilled from the wound. Having a baby is always a little messy, and a good abdominal toilet at the end of the operation is essential.

At this point I delivered the repaired womb out of the tummy in order to demonstrate to the cameras beyond all doubt that there were no Fallopian tubes present. The womb was replaced, the peritoneum closed, and the wound stitched up in layers. The saline drip in the back of Lesley's hand was replaced by a blood drip, previously prepared in readiness. Next day she would feel very little discomfort and would not be lacking in a sense of well being thanks to that litre of blood transfusion. How different from the feeling of drainage and exhaustion if that fluid and blood loss had not been replaced.

12.05 a.m. The operation was over and I was able to attend to the scene beyond the table. Baby Brown had been weighed naked, 5 lb. 12 oz., and wrapped up again. She had been crying loudly most of the time. Don Hilson announced that she was absolutely normal and in fine condition, so I was handed the infant for a few moments. A jubilant Bob and Jean joined me, and I passed Louise, as she was to be named, to Bob. It was his brain, skill and perseverance and Jean's hard-working devotion which had led to this wonderful moment of achievement. We stood briefly together for the cameras to preserve the moment and then returned Louise to her cot and her guardian nurses.

Meanwhile John Brown sat with Sheena in Lesley's hospital room, talking about how lucky he was to have been able to come to Oldham. A sister burst in excitedly.

'You may go and see your baby daughter now. A porter will take you along. Lesley's fine.'

'What did you say, sister?'

'You may go to see your baby daughter as soon as the porter arrives.'

Sheena later told me how John was speechless. Tears poured down his face. He stood up and banged his clenched fist against the wall. When he regained control, he kissed sister, kissed my wife, who was also now happily weeping, and ran out of the room. He ran all the way downstairs along the sixty yards of corridor to the operating theatre, pursued by the porter and by Sheena. Senior police officers were grouped round the door with Fred Baxter. Doors opened into a long green corridor. There we stood with Louise's cot on a trolley. The baby was lifted into John's arms.

'I can't believe it! I can't believe it!' he cried out. 'I don't know what to say.'

He gazed mesmerized at the infant, until someone gently guided the baby back into the cot. Lesley was still peacefully asleep – unable to join in the happy delirium all around. The baby was whisked up to the special care unit. Don Hilson and I put together a statement to be issued immediately to the Press Association announcing the birth. Louise was healthy and normal, and she was beautiful too, really lovely.

Lesley soon recovered from the anaesthetic, but after arousal passed into a pleasant sleep. She was wheeled from the recovery area back to her room. Blood pressure and pulse were normal, the womb well contracted with little loss from it. While she slept the blood slowly dripped into her veins.

For me exhaustion now set in, but we decided to telephone the good news to my son, and then Bob took over the lines to let everyone know of the happy news. Sheena and I drove home through the quiet streets feeling relaxed and tranquil at last. We took the telephone off the receiver as soon as we arrived, and sleep followed within minutes of hitting the sheets. But it was impossible to resist the radio news at 7.30 the next morning and the programme called 'What the Papers Say'. So we were hardly refreshed after only six hours' sleep. At 8.30 a.m. I re-connected the telephone and rang the hospital for a report about Lesley and the baby. Both were fine, and Louise had already taken some fluid by mouth.

Breakfast followed, with a brief look at the morning paper. Then I drove to the hospital. Many newspaper men still hung about, and the first question asked was, 'How's the baby?'

'Fine,' I said. 'You must wait for the official statement for anything more, but this will soon be announced.'

Lesley was awake, bathed and propped up in bed. The blood drip had been replaced by a simple normal saline. Every system was normal, so we stopped the drip and removed the needle. She had already taken some sweet tea.

'Can I see baby?' she enquired.

'Yes. I'll go and bring her now,' I promised.

I made my way to the special ward, and I was delighted to be greeted by the paediatricians with the news that Louise was well, normal, and could leave the unit straight away to join her mother. I was deeply touched when all of them, including the paediatric nurses, insisted that I should be the one to give Lesley her baby.

We covered the trolley cot with a white shawl, and off we went – down the lift, along the corridor and up to the third floor of the Maternity Block. No one disturbed our little procession. The screen guarding Lesley's bed from the doorway was still in position. We wheeled the cot behind the screen unseen from the bed.

'Lesley,' I said, 'we've brought your baby. She's going to stay with you.'

Sister handed me the baby behind the screen. I carried the infant to the foot of the bed, then leaned over to place her in Lesley's arms. Everyone had slipped out quietly. Like her husband earlier Lesley was speechless, but her expression was so moving, her look so eloquent that words were unnecessary. She cradled the infant and then managed to whisper, 'Thank you for my baby. Thank you.'

Louise Joy had arrived, a whole new person to make this family complete at long last. I doubt if I shall ever share such a moment in my life again.

26
Farewell to Oldham
Robert Edwards

Our work at Kershaw's was ending. We had taken in a final group of patients and a fourth wonderful pregnancy began. So hostile scientists could hardly carp now about the efficacy of our technique – one baby, Louise, a lovely girl born and thriving, and three more children on the way.

With many regrets and farewells Jean and I prepared to quit. We were bringing down the shutters on ten years of our lives. We were not the only ones preparing to leave. Our last patients were carrying their suitcases out of the hospital even as we were packing up our equipment. Mr Holmes, too, was retiring. It was the end of an episode for all of us.

Anyway we had done it: a grandstand finish just as Patrick had to retire from the National Health Service. It would not, of course, be the end of our fruitful collaboration. For the moment we had no facilities to continue our work but somehow, somewhere, not too far from Cambridge, we would begin again. I could not help but think of the money we had refused from competing newspapers and TV networks. That finance could have helped our work to continue without interruption.

Just before the birth of Louise I had been astonished to receive a visitor who wished to give me a considerable sum of money in exchange for the story of our work. He had been followed by others with the same request: we had become a valuable business proposition to British and foreign newspapers, magazines and television networks. The amounts offered were scarcely credible – a quarter of a million pounds became the lowest figure mentioned. I had virtually thrown the first pressman out of my laboratory because the whole situation seemed to me ludicrous. But they were all in deadly earnest; one after the other they joined in the bidding, each one making a more ridiculous (better!)

offer. There had even been suggestions that the money be paid quietly into a foreign bank, tax free – or that a prize could be offered but it would be fixed. We had felt very virtuous turning down sums, fantastic sums in seven figures – but we felt confident that eventually public sources would finance our future work. It seems to us now that our confidence then was misplaced.

When we returned to Cambridge we waited for news of our three pregnancies. Louise flourished. Forty-one different investigations had been carried out by the paediatricians, all of them demonstrating what we already knew – that Louise was an absolutely normal child.

But two of the three foetuses growing in their mothers' wombs were, alas, to meet with disaster. One was lost a few weeks after the embryo had been implanted – it had been a perfectly normal foetus but triploid with sixty-nine chromosomes. How ironic that that should have occurred when all those years earlier we had discovered no triploids in any of the tiny cleaving embryos.

The other foetus had an even more tragic end, miles from our care, far away in the Yorkshire Dales. More than half way through the pregnancy – at twenty-and-a-half weeks to be precise – when every test had been successfully completed, a crisis arose during a holiday in the Pennines. Our patient, aware that a miscarriage might be impending, hastened to the nearby Airedale General Hospital. Despite all care and attention the baby was lost – an immature boy weighing only 800 grams who lived only for an hour or so. A few weeks more within the mother's womb and the baby boy would have had a fighting chance for he was fully normal in every way. Patrick tried to console our unlucky patient. She had been infertile for ten years. She had lost both tubes and one ovary. Our method had been the only chance she had of ever becoming pregnant. And though her eventual pregnancy had not concluded happily as we had all hoped and expected, she determined to try again once we resumed our work in the future.

Our fourth baby was born in Stobhill Hospital in Glasgow in January 1979, under the care of the patient's local gynaecologist who had originally referred her to us. Our patient went into labour a little early – the baby was not expected until February. The weather that January had been appalling. Snow fell upon snow upon snow. There were massive drifts and news of lorries and cars abandoned on the roads which overnight were very soon buried under the latest heavy snowfall. The road conditions were such that we did not arrive in time for the birth. When Patrick reached the Glasgow hospital the delivery had taken place one hour earlier. No matter – though we were not there to welcome the healthy baby boy it was as marvellous and happy an occasion as the birth of Louise had been. Alastair – for that was his name – Alastair has grown and flourished normally ever since.

That same arctic winter month Patrick and I presented details of our work at the Royal College of Obstetricians and Gynaecologists in London. It was a crowded meeting and we were startled and heartened by the standing ovation we were given at its end. It is a wonderful feeling, as Patrick has said, to receive the warm approval of distinguished colleagues and experts. The Secretary of the College told us that such an ovation had not occurred ever before in the whole history of the College.

Patrick escaped our miserable weather the next month when he flew to San Francisco for the American Fertility Society's annual meeting. It had been planned that he would give there an even more detailed presentation of our work. I was somewhat envious of Patrick enjoying Californian sunny days as we slithered on ice in Cambridge, where bursting pipes made plumbers the heroes of the day.

But I was warmed in my own way when I heard how Patrick was received. The American Fertility Society had presented him with a special plaque of commendation and his lecture had been listened to raptly by over 1000 people, who not only crowded the seats of the huge hall but filled the doorways and corridors outside it. Patrick told me how the ovation at the end of his lecture on this occasion had almost moved him to tears. Such warmth touches me too – for we have had many jagged criticisms hurled at us both, some of which have been frankly tinged with jealousy and prejudice. It is nice to receive occasional compliments from valued colleagues.

Our pleasure in our success was tempered however by the fact that a request for State funds to be made available in Cambridge could not be granted. We could have a special unit in Manchester all right, but there were insufficient hospital facilities in Cambridge. It was time to look for alternative possibilities. We could only develop things satisfactorily together in or near Cambridge.

Patrick and I still have work to do together. There is a very long list of patients who have been referred to us in good faith by gynaecologists and other doctors. These couples may not only be helped themselves, but in their turn, as we develop the method further and modify and probably improve it, they may help many other women; for the work is still at its relatively early stages.

Meanwhile other professional units and centres with interest in the work we have started are being set up in the United Kingdom, and abroad. The Ethical Committee advising the Health, Education and Welfare Department of the USA recommended the use of federal funds for research in our field. And very active groups in Australia, especially in Melbourne, pursued and are pursuing our objectives. Preliminary plans are also being made in various European countries and in Japan.

We continue to receive hundreds of letters from gynaecologists and doctors the world over requesting treatment for their patients. Many of the stories are sad, even pathetic, others are occasionally ridiculous and Patrick naturally finds it painful to have to disillusion patients who have not fully understood the implications of our work. It was embarrassing, for instance, for him to have to disillusion the occasional lady several years past her menopause that there was no chance of her becoming pregnant.

What of the future? What are the implications of this work all over the world? Patrick writes: 'Of the future one can hope that there will be a steady increase of knowledge of fertilization, of early growth of the embryo and reimplantation, so that an increasing number of sterile women will be able to have the opportunity to bear a child. The progress will be slow but it will probably be sure and effective.'

I think, frankly, that we have brought hope to thousands of couples and interest to millions of others watching from the sidelines. The new advances we have made in the treatment of infertility are perhaps sufficient in themselves, sufficient reward for all our efforts. We must improve our success rate though, make our work more realistic for the hundreds of patients on our waiting lists. If we can do this we shall be able to replace many current methods of treating infertility – especially those requiring extensive surgery with only a slight chance of pregnancy. Many gynaecologists will be trained in our methods so that they in turn can help their own patients.

The cure of certain kinds of infertility is not the only advance we now have within our grasp. There are so many other opportunities. We have the chance to look at the causes of some other human disorders – those upsets where the smallest change in the number of chromosomes in a foetus can disastrously affect its future well-being. We are all familiar with Mongolism but there are also other disorders – in sexual development and other conditions leading to mental retardation. I still believe that the secrets of the causes of these disorders lie in those ripening eggs, in those chromosomes moving so steadily through the egg as it undergoes its ripening process. We can turn to a closer examination of these problems.

These are wonderful opportunities which, if successful, can alleviate, indeed prevent, much human suffering. Even so, there are other major advances to be made, other challenges elsewhere. I often think of that embryo which grew for nine days in our culture, of how it wriggled out of its membrane and expanded beautifully. Consider again that embryo: within it all the stem cells of the body's organs were differentiating and growing, appearing steadily one by one. This, for me, was excitement magnified because it offered all the beginnings of human embryology to us; here was the chance of watching and analysing the appearances and growth of the different tissues of the body – the heart, the blood system, the brain. These tissues could one day form in front of our very eyes!

These embryonic cells contain mysteries that can and must be solved – how they increase rapidly and then successively grow into different organs during early growth. And most exciting of all, they may possibly be used in treating many human disorders.

We need more knowledge of these very early stages if we are to discover how it is that illnesses such as German measles or drugs such as thalidomide interfere with normal development. Perhaps we can find some clues, however small, if we observe the growing sensitivity and susceptibility to such harmful agents of cells growing in the embryo in culture. Perhaps we shall be able to understand why other embryos succumb and become invasive to their own mother, threatening her by their massive, disordered challenge. Any knowledge along these lines, however meagre, would be a help.

Will we be able to discover how these cells appear and develop so regularly? Will we be able to extract the stem cells of various organs from the embryo, the precious foundation cells of all the body's organs and then use them therapeutically? Will it ever be possible to use these cells to correct deficiencies in other human beings – to replace one deficient tissue with another that functions normally? For instance, will we be able to use the blood-forming cells of an embryo to re-colonize defective blood-forming tissue in an adult or child? And will these notions be met with pursed lips and frowning faces?

Perhaps the whole concept will fall to the ground and be proved to be a mistaken one in medical treatment. I doubt it. So much is on our side – the very foundation cells have been and will be again in our cultures and we know they are capable of displaying the initial signs of tissue differentiation. These same embryonic cells may offer us one further therapeutic advantage. They may one day be used without having to worry about graft rejection such as we all know is associated with kidney, heart and liver transplantations.

Perhaps this whole approach may seem heartless to those who feel that the embryo is a human being who must be protected at all costs. I cannot share this opinion. If we can alleviate certain disorders in children or adults who are suffering greatly or who may be dying, then surely we must be allowed to use these cells, taken from an embryo while still only the size of a pinhead – stem cells collected and grown in our cultures until they can be used to repair damage or defect.

To grow foetuses to later stages of growth when they take a recognizable human shape and then extract their organs would be utterly wrong and is a repugnant concept; but to obtain cell colonies from minute embryos useful in medicine for the alleviation of certain human disorders – is that not a legitimate target to aim at? It is a target that may be reached, should be reached, if we can understand the priceless secrets of those embryonic cells growing in our cultures.

We know that our work is opening new horizons in human reproduction – indeed, it has already opened some. We are aware, too, that it introduces the possibility of genetic engineering or embryological engineering in one form or another, as feared by those correspondents ten years ago when we first began our work. Now that we have demonstrated that human conception can occur outside the human body, many investigations can be done which were impossible before. These are challenges which we should not fear, though we must be on our guard against abuses.

Science moves haphazardly and often unpredictably. Yet what is merely a gleam in the eye of a research scientist today may be familiar to everyone tomorrow. There can be no excuse for manipulating human characteristics unnecessarily and cloning is an extreme form of manipulation – a needless and unattractive exercise in genetic engineering designed to replace one person by another. But perhaps even this technique may be utilized eventually for the benefit of humanity in directions which we do not apprehend today, such as averting the rejection of transplanted embryonic cells. Each new discovery should be examined dispassionately and its benefits weighed in the balance. Such is the nature of collaboration between science and medicine.